CONTENTS

LIST OF EXERCISES

PREFACE

So many different health care workers offer health care: ambulance workers, specialists, speech therapists, optometrists, physiotherapists, general practitioners (GPs), dentists, rehabilitation counsellors, nurses, occupational therapists, pharmacists, radiologists, laboratory scientists, medical records and health administrators, and many others. They are all are an essential part of our health system. This book delves into health care ethics from the starting point of the workplace, the training ground for health care workers. It is designed to be useful to all health care workers.

This book is about ethics. You don't need to be an ethicist to understand ethics in the health context, and you don't need to have learnt a lot of philosophy to be able to think about ethics as you work in your health profession. This book is written so that the information in it can be used in a practical way in your everyday work. It starts with you, the professional carer, and examines the way professional work and your interaction with your clients or patients is shaped by ethics.

Ethics is, after all, only a tool. It is not just an abstract introspective pursuit. Rather, it helps us reflect on real life issues, and is also a process that can be applied to real concerns and real situations as they unfold. Ethics in health contexts is sometimes simply called 'ethics'; at other times it is called 'bioethics', or 'medical ethics'. You may like to choose a definition of ethics that you understand best from the following options:
- ethics—'ways of understanding and examining the moral life'.[1]
- bioethics—'a popular contraction for "biomedical ethics", which is the study of moral value in the life sciences and in their clinical application'.[2]
- medical ethics—'the analytical activity in which the concepts, assumptions, beliefs, attitudes, emotion, reasons, and arguments underlying medico-moral decision making are examined critically'.[3]

The common theme followed in this book is that health care ethics is not only about setting acceptable standards, but is also about reflecting on what you should aim for in your work as health care professionals. It is about reflecting on optimal standards, and pursuing those standards. The book is written in an interactive way. Dotted throughout, you will find individual and group exercises that will help you think about particular issues or standards, or particular styles of ethical reflection. Tutorial-type triggers and case studies are also included.

While there is a section on ethics theories at the end of the book, in Chapter 10, you will find ethics theories and frameworks woven into all the other chapters. As you work through the exercises, you will become more familiar with key ways of identifying, and working to resolve, ethics issues in health care. In this framework, the philosophical aspect of ethics becomes a tool that you, as a health care worker, can use to reflect on ethics as it applies in your profession and in your clinical work.

You will not be an expert in ethics after working through this book, but you will be considerably more informed. You will naturally want to consult with other colleagues who are interested in ethics, and with ethicists, at times when you are faced with complex challenges. This book starts you on a path of ethical reflection. It also encourages you to consult with others so that you do not face ethical challenges, as a health care worker, alone. The author, Catherine Berglund (BSc (Psychol) PhD (Community Med)) is not a practising health professional. Yet, with undergraduate psychology training, and postgraduate research and health ethics experience, she is often asked to advise on reflection processes for health professionals.

This text meets the need to consider ethics in the routine context of health care. It follows a sequence that is familiar in health care education and practice: training, adopting a profession, becoming a team member in a health care setting, beginning to see clients, and working with clients as their treatment progresses.

The book also meets the need to learn about ethics theory. But it moves beyond the traditional theory-oriented structure of most ethics texts, to a structure that is generated by practical, professional, and client needs. Key doctrines, moral distinctions, and theories are woven into the text. Principlist approaches are explored, as are frameworks such as utilitarianism and deontology. The text does not favour any one of these. Rather, it leaves the choice up to the reader. Readers are encouraged to relate the ideas presented to their own views and experiences, and to answer questions as they read.

This text takes a novel approach to teaching ethics, drawing on practical experience and contemporary issues in its exploration of ethical choices made in health care. Taking the sequence described above—training, adoption of a profession, becoming a team member, seeing and working with clients—the book focuses on the interaction between the health provider and his or her client.

Teachers of health care ethics can use this book as a training manual or class resource. It provides an extensive choice of tutorial triggers, and contains sufficient theory to be able to be used in an ethics curriculum, or integrated with core health care subjects.

Notes

1   R. Gillon, *Philosophical Medical Ethics*, John Wiley & Sons, Chichester, United Kingdom, 1986, p. 2.
2   J. D. Moreno, *Deciding Together: Bioethics and Moral Consensus*, Oxford University Press, New York, 1995, p. 4.
3   Gillon, p. 2.

ACKNOWLEDGMENTS

I feel privileged to have had the opportunity to learn from many people during the preparation of this book. Some are learned writers and colleagues, others are patients or health care professionals, and some are friends and family. Many have prompted me to begin this project by their writings, others by their spoken word, and others have encouraged and supported me throughout. I owe them my deepest gratitude and give my heartfelt thanks to them all.

The support of Oxford University Press in the writing and production of this book has been superb—I would particularly like to thank Jill Henry and Michele Sabto, for support during the first edition preparation, and Debra James for support during the second edition preparation.

For my daughters, Vivienne and Ellen

ABBREVIATIONS

ACTG	AIDS Clinical Trials Group (USA)
AGPS	Australian Government Publishing Service
AIDS	acquired immune deficiency syndrome
AMA	Australian Medical Association
CHF	Consumers' Health Forum
CPR	cardiopulmonary resuscitation
DNR	Do Not Resuscitate
HIV	human immunodeficiency virus
HREC	human research ethics committee
IEC	institutional ethics committee
IVF	in vitro fertilisation
NHMRC	National Health and Medical Research Council
QA	quality assurance
QALY	quality-adjusted life year
SARS	severe acute respiratory syndrome
TGA	Therapeutic Goods Administration
WHO	World Health Organization

1

Caring as professionals

Overview

- Becoming a professional carer
- Professional goals and duties
- Professional guidelines on ethics
- Caring in multidisciplinary teams

This first chapter identifies ethics in practice, for individual carers and groups of carers. Personal and professional bounds and ideals are explored. Ethics is explained as an optimal standard of thought and action. Training and role boundaries are discussed, and broad beneficence issues are canvassed.

BECOMING A PROFESSIONAL CARER

Becoming a professional carer is not an easy decision. It can take years to decide which profession to choose. People are often asked, as they approach their final years of school, 'What do you want to do?'. Think back to when you started your training. This might be when you left school, or it might be later. Why did you choose to train in your health profession? Did you hold certain values and ideals of caring, or was it something else that prompted you to choose your profession?

Education selection specialists (people who advise students on careers and courses, or who advise institutions on which students to accept) know that there is more to being a successful and productive professional health care worker than academic marks. Increasingly, they are searching for those with the capacity to work with others, to reflect on difficult problems, to make a virtue of wanting to care, to serve, and to go beyond self-needs to meet the needs of others. They are interested in why people want to become health carers, rather than in any superior intellectual capability of remembering facts and performing certain procedural skills. In other words, they are looking at the person who will be carrying out the work, not just at their narrowly defined 'technical' ability to do the work.

Ethics, as it is understood in this book, takes as its starting point the fact that, first and foremost, you are an individual. You were a unique individual before you began your training, you are an individual at work, where you are also a health care worker, and you are an individual outside work. There are very different people in this world, and one of the things that distinguishes us from each other is the way we choose to live our lives. Given that you bring much of yourself to your work, it is worthwhile thinking about the sort of person you are before we begin our discussion of 'professional' ethics.

Take a minute to think about how you live your life. Try and identify, in your own words, one fundamental principle in the way you live your life, and in the way you live alongside others.

Many of the philosophers whose work we draw on in professional ethics actually wrote more about individual ethics (that is, about the ethics of decisions made by individuals) than about group standards or norms. Philosophers thought about how we should live our lives and relate to others. They thought about the structure of our society; about what we, as individuals, owe to our society; and about what we can, and should, expect in return. They thought also about our higher duties to God. Nowadays, religion is often separated from professional ethics, but if it is a large part of how you live your life, it would be artificial for you to do that. You will see comments and exercises from many of these early philosophers dotted throughout the book. Try this one now.

When you think about how you try to live, think about the virtue you aspire to. What is that virtue? How would you define it, and how do you know if you have achieved it?

The key feature of Socrates' discussions was the way in which participants were encouraged to elicit and question beliefs. Some of the central values that Socrates espoused were justice, courage, and pity.[1] He tried to define them through reflection and discussion, like the reflection you just undertook for yourself. This reflection process is appropriate for our professional lives too. Justice and courage may be listed as two of the modern nurse's virtues, as nurses advance their clients' interests and attempt to maximise the autonomy of their clients.[2]

Our values form our ethics standards and they determine what we expect from others. In some ethics frameworks, virtue and the formation of central values is paramount. There is a sense of a moral self-development. We probably apply this notion of moral self-development, without thinking about it, in our own lives. We do not, for instance, expect children to be rational and moral in the way in which they relate to others and the world because we know that some of this is learnt. We gradually teach them what is expected, what we value, and what we hope that they will value. As they grow older, they begin to recognise, in abstract, that it is not just the fact that these values are advocated by parents and guardians that makes them desirable as guides for life. They come to value these virtues themselves.

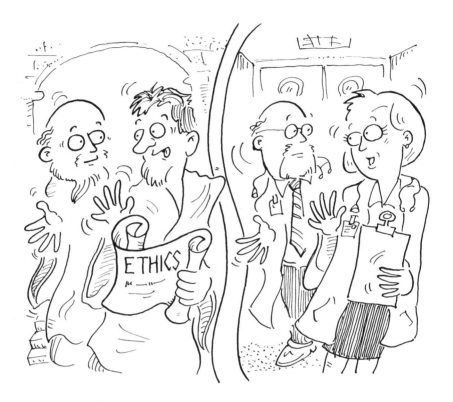

In ancient Greece and Rome, there were designated forums for debating what was right and virtuous, and for reasoning why that was so. Learned people were trained to reflect and to hold monologues or debates challenging others to refine their thoughts, actions, and reasoning. Socrates and Plato led this tradition, and there was an expectation that people who rose to prominence in society would learn to reflect and debate personal and social ethics. Plato was Socrates' student and Aristotle's teacher. Plato emphasised that winning a debate was not the purpose of the discussion. The purpose was to search for the truth.[3]

When a person becomes a member of a profession, they become one of the people who help define the ideals of the profession. They bring their own ethics to the profession, and their ethics are influenced by what others have defined as appropriate ethical standards for that profession. It is a fluid process of sharing thoughts, and of learning to work together towards common goods. (Bear in mind that the word 'good' is used as a noun here, that it is a thing or concept, not an adjective.) The process of reflecting on professional caring, of identifying important aspects of caring, and of debating what professionals should aim for continues the tradition of ancient debates, albeit in a different guise. You may like to consider whether you care enough about your ideals to defend them against others. In professional debates, we would do well to remember to keep discussion constructive, as is urged in Plato's tradition, and not simply use ethics as a tool to score points off our colleagues. The reflection process is more important than keeping score.

What you have done so far is to start to reflect on what you value, how you live, what you strive for, and how your values are part of the way you live up to your professional responsibilities. Personal reflection on professional responsibilities has become integrated with health care, and health care ethics is generally seen as a modern phenomenon. Much has been written about the fact that technological innovation and development in health care has led to an exponential increase in ethics dilemmas, and many of those involved in health care wonder if and how we should put such advances to use.[4] Medicine and health care presents such ethically stark issues that it is very useful to use ethics as a tool to unravel the issues and work out, in a reasoned fashion, what to do when faced with those issues in practice. On the other hand, even before great technological advances, the daily aspects of health care were the subject of ethics reflection. It may just be that, now that technology (including technology associated with health care) has such a high profile, ethics also has a higher profile.

You could think about ethics in health care as really being about three things: individual ethics and values, group ethics and values, and professional ethics and values. Writers in health care ethics vary in their approach. Some concentrate on individual virtue, others on group notions of ethics, or on philosophical analysis of ethical stances and values. This book gives you a wide range of exercises to do on your own or in groups so that you can experiment with those approaches. All of the approaches share a common purpose: to assist health care workers to make ethical decisions, and to monitor their own and others' practices so that the health care process is 'ethically aware'. They also potentially assist the people planning and receiving services. Ethics is becoming a joint effort, and reflection on ethics is increasingly consultative. More on this is included in Chapter 7.

The following exercise asks you to think about the values and ideals that you held at an early stage of your health care training. It has been adapted from a reflective exercise written by Ken Cox for a jointly authored distance-education course on clinical ethics.[5] Think about when you were just beginning training, when you were just beginning to learn to be a health care professional. You might like to look back to photos of yourself when you were beginning training to jog your memory.

Exercise 1.1 Ideals and values

Write down the words that spring to mind about your images of yourself and your ideals and values as a beginning clinical student.

....

....

....

....

....

....

....

....

....

....

It is part of reality that ideals, values, and circumstances can conflict. From your list, strike out the ideals that you no longer hold; write down what changed your values; and add some new values. More importantly, think about what might have reinforced or changed your values.

Looking at your list of current ideals and values, do you think you are ethical? Do you have the potential to act ethically as a health care professional if you implement those ideals?

Ethics is more than an expression of what might be. It is more than writing down what we agree with, or what we think we should aim for. Learning to be a professional is also about learning skills, and about becoming able to put those skills into action. We learn to put our ethics or ideals into action too. The skills aspect of professional work is inextricably linked to professional ethics. As Pellegrino has stated, the ethics of a profession is not 'the norms actually followed by professionals, or the professional codes they espouse, but rather the moral obligations deductible from the kinds of activity in which they are engaged'.[6] So, your individual natures, and the skills you learn, are intertwined in your sense of professional ethics.

This is just starting to be recognised by teachers of health care ethics around the world. They are increasingly stepping away from the dramatic bioethics dilemmas, and the purely philosophical discussion, and are beginning, instead, to bring ethics back into our everyday lives, helping us to acknowledge its existence in everyday health situations.[7] That is the approach of this book. You need to be constantly re-examining your list of ideals and values, and as your list of professional skills and types of professional activities grows, you should be thinking about how you should act. You need, in other words, to think about ethics in your every-day work.

While wanting to care for others is a common reason for becoming a health care worker, the decision about what type of health profession to join is much more complex. What skills you might be good at should be considered. If you are making this decision, you need to ask yourself what sort of work do health care workers in a particular field really do, and what sort of work would you enjoy? Career counsellors, or seeing health care in action, will help you to decide.

Work experience can help too. Many budding health professionals take on part-time work in health contexts, and this exposes them to a variety of health care work, and to the reality of the day-to-day aspects of health care. When I was at university, doing an undergraduate psychology degree, I worked in a kitchen of a large private hospital. I learnt a lot, saw a range of health professionals in action and in the wards, and I got a feel for how health care was being practised in that hospital. I learnt that the ethic of caring extends not only to medical staff and other health profes-sionals, but also to the auxiliary staff. They are all part of a health team. The ethic of caring is warmer in an institution in which that is acknowl-edged at all levels. We regularly took the time to stop and chat to patients as we delivered their meals, if they initiated conversation. Some patients became very friendly; they and we looked forward to us popping in for a hello or a chat. If patients obviously needed privacy, we respected that, and we learnt to be as discreet as possible in delivering and collecting trays. When people felt more ill than usual, we would try to substitute more easily eaten food (after checking with the dietitian and ward staff of course), and if they just had an appetite for something else, we tried to accommodate that. We learnt to respond to needs and wishes, to behave with respect and courtesy, and to work smoothly as a team so that there was maximum service and caring. 'Providing care', and 'providing it caringly' may be subtly different. The ethic of caring is not just about technical application of skill; it is also about how that skill is applied.

Think about the first time you felt the ethic of caring, and make a note of it. Also, think about how non-health care professionals show this ethic where you work.

The process of learning, and the awareness of the culture of caring, continues throughout professional life. It starts very early. Your own early learning should be recognised, even if it appears to be less glamorous than 'real' health care or 'real' professional work. You perhaps learn as fast in your early work, as you do in your later years as senior, or more qualified, health care workers.

The professional training system is openly acknowledged to be a slow process. It takes time to accumulate knowledge and skill. And it takes time to gather insight into proper standards. Our society acknowledges that it is necessary to fund training through public taxes. We have teaching hospitals, which are centres of excellence, and which strive to train others in that excellence. Teaching hospitals work in partnership with colleges and universities to train a skilled and experienced workforce. Our system lets students and juniors 'do' health work under supervision, and by applying less rigorous skill standards to them (in the presence of a trained person to support, supervise, and back the student up), allows them the freedom to learn. As their skill and knowledge level increases, students do increasingly difficult tasks under decreasing supervision. The professional skill is slowly transferred from supervisor to student. The professional power and discretion to decide the 'right' manner in achieving that work is also slowly transferred. This happens in professional ethics too. Through mentoring, academic instruction, role modelling, group discussion, and other systems, we gradually form the 'moral professional', and we trust that by the time students graduate, they have sufficient understanding of standards in the profession.

Exercise 1.2 Skills and limits

Think about one professional standard that you have learnt. Make a note of how and when you learnt it, and when you first put it into action.

....

....

....

....

....

....

....

....

....

....

You may have chosen a level of knowledge (or practical skill), or you may have chosen a standard that is more about the way that skill is delivered. Learning increasingly difficult and finely tuned professional standards is part of becoming a professional carer. We learn, in fine detail, what the job is, and how we are expected to do it.

When you are trained as a professional, you acquire the privileged knowledge of that profession. You will continue to learn throughout your professional life, constantly updating or extending your knowledge and skill base. Part of being a professional is this commitment to keep learning, to continually strive to be able to deliver the best possible care for your clients. The flipside of this is that there are limits to your knowledge and skill. You need to have insight into how knowledgeable and capable you are. There is a danger for others if you think that you are much more skilled than you actually are, and you go beyond your safe limits in dealing with people. This reflection on and insight into skill and knowledge is essential. Practising insight into your skill level actually provides you with a model for reflecting on your ethical limits. Think of a skill that you are still learning, and try the following exercise.

My safe limits in performing the skill are:

....

....

....

....

....

....

....

My judgement of my safe limit is based on:

....

....

....

....

....

....

....

The consequences of exceeding this limit for the client are:

....

....

....

....

....

....

....

....

Recognising your limits in skill is very helpful because it starts you off on self-reflection, and on reflecting on all aspects of health care. Reflection is a key part of ethics. It should continue throughout your career.

Life-long commitment is not uncommon in professions. Historically, people entered the equivalent of holy orders to receive the depth of training that was required, and they often pledged themselves to the ideals of learning and service. To have a profession was, literally, to have professed oaths, such as obedience to church values, honesty, and high standards of service.[8] This is similar to the intensity of devotion and long apprenticeship that a successful professional still needs today. There are still professional ideals that are avowed by particular health care professions. These ideals go beyond a particular duty to an employer or contract of employment. Once professed, they apply wherever that professional works. Professionals have an ongoing duty to consider appropriate moral or ethical standards, and to reflect on their own behaviour.

PROFESSIONAL GOALS AND DUTIES

By definition, professional work is skilled, and is done to benefit others. The community trusts that proper standards are applied in carrying out that work. You need to be familiar with the extent of your skills, and by carrying out that skill properly, which includes doing it competently and ethically, you fulfil the trust placed in you. Just as the community places its trust in you so too you trust others to carry out work involving skills different to your own.

Proper standards, of course, need definition. Professions, by their very nature, have a responsibility to define what their goals are; the expected role, and corresponding duties, of practitioners; and the limits of the service they can be expected to provide.

Goals are something to aspire to; they are the ethically optimal position. In contrast, duties are something we are obliged to fulfil. It is a minimal position to only fulfil strict duties without aspiring to higher goals. Virtue is receiving renewed attention in modern ethics texts, incorporating the Aristotelian notion of ideals. The motivation towards ethical action, as well as achievement of ethical actions, is reflected on. Some people, who accept special roles, like health care professionals, can assume certain higher responsibilities than others. Then, they are expected to exceed normal moral requirements towards what would be regarded as moral ideals and excellence in others.[9] Basic duties can translate into lists of duties, or obligations, and prohibitions, all of which are outlined for you before you start working in your profession. The first documentation you might see when starting a new job is a 'statement of duties', or a general job description that implies duties. These vary widely between professions because of the different skills and corresponding responsibilities involved in that profession. They also vary between different units or specialisations within that profession because of the different services those units provide.

Do either of the following sets of tasks, associated with the jobs of occupational therapist and registered nurse respectively, come close to the basic duties of your job?
- *An occupational therapist helps 'mentally, physically, developmentally, or emotionally disabled individuals develop, recover, or maintain daily living and work skills'.[10] Occupational therapists will often be assigned, in their duties, to individuals in one particular age group or disability, and will be required to design programs that assist with day-to-day life skills.*
- *A registered nurse is required to 'observe, assess, and record symptoms, reactions, and progress; administer medications; assist in convalescence and rehabilitation; instruct patients and their families in proper care; and help individuals and groups take steps to improve and maintain their health'.[11] The level of responsibility varies with experience.*

Care to self is also a responsibility: to keep oneself safe and well, and then set about the duties of helping others. Codes of practice, and the ideals they profess, are there to encourage optimal behaviour, and serve as a safeguard to ensure that certain basic standards of behaviour are adhered to, and that professionals are committed to offering proper quality of care. Registration bodies are established to make sure that only those people who are trained and are currently competent to practise in health care do so. When you enter your profession, you effectively agree to meet the standards of professional behaviour expected of you. Formal registration makes this clearer. Your professional body then fully expects your approach and conduct to be competent and ethical. Your peers, in effect, expect you to uphold professional standards. If standards are breached to a significant extent, professional bodies may take the step of deregistering professionals. This is effectively a statement that the standard of care offered by that professional is deficient. This assessment as to the standard of care can be made in relation to ethics as well as practical skill. These professional regulatory mechanisms are further discussed in Chapter 8. If people who purport to be professionally trained are not, then we become worried. Consider the example from Buenos Aires of an Argentinean man with no medical degree, who worked as a neurologist in a major hospital for sixteen years, chaired a specialist conference, and co-wrote a book on medicine. Described as 'a great seducer with the gift of the gab', and both brilliant and a psychopath, he was subsequently charged with forgery, false exercise of a profession, and causing serious injury after a woman told police she had suffered brain damage in an operation he recommended.[12]

We are worried about such people because they have not gone through the training of the profession, nor are they subject to the same degree of rigorous peer review and sanction as member professionals are.

Dr Jack Kevorkian, the American doctor who promoted his 'suicide machine' as an option for terminally ill patients, also troubled professional medical practitioners. Even apart from the arguments of whether suicide, professionally assisted or not, was ethical (and this will be discussed further in Chapter 6), Dr Kevorkian was retired from medical practice. He was once a registered pathologist, but when he allegedly started assisting people in their requested suicides, he was no longer practising. He was, in effect, beyond professional sanction, but was still using his title of doctor.[13] Dr Kevorkian's actions have attracted significant media attention, and he has been tried in a number of criminal courts in the USA. You may like to further consider the border between ethics and law. It is covered in Chapter 8.

Similarly, practitioners who work alone for a long period of time are disproportionately the focus of disciplinary and remedial practice programs. An extreme example is that of the English GP, Dr Harold Shipman, who was convicted in 2000 of murdering fifteen patients. The GP had a long-term pattern of working alone and making unannounced home visits. The unusual dress of many of his patients in day clothes (whereas people who feel ill are normally lying in bed in pyjamas), and sometimes in a seated position, at the time of their death were noticed by a local undertaker. Then, a local GP expressed concern about the rate of death certificates she was being asked to countersign, prompting an initial police investigation, which was completed without specific conclusion. The possibly fraudulent inclusion of his name as a beneficiary in a will prompted the eventual successful criminal investigation.[14] Audits of his patient files and deaths of other patients led to calls for further charges.[15] Commentary from the UK focused on concern that the activities were not detected sooner, and restoring the public trust in the quality and appropriateness and accountability of professional medical services.[16]

Opportunities for detection are highest when individual actions and judgements are accountable to others. This was emphasised by the Shipman Inquiry chairman Dame Janet Smith in her lengthy findings into the practice and death certification process. In the Inquiry, Dame Smith found that over 200 patients had been killed.[17]

Exercise 1.3 Responsibility and accountability

Try the following exercise. Look through the suggested process for certification of a death in England, as in the Shipman Inquiry Report (in Third Report, at pp. 496–510), and write them out again as a series of steps. Then, circle the steps in the process that set out who are the appropriate people to undertake responsibilities in certifying and checking circumstances of each person's death, and those which link the opinion of individuals to the scrutiny of others. This is to build in accountability. Consider who is undertaking each responsibility and who their accountability is to.

Form 1 is to be completed by a health professional (doctor, nurse, or paramedic) to confirm the fact of death, the circumstances of death, those present, and their contact details. An external examination of the body is undertaken, and findings recorded. This form is transmitted to the coroner's office.

Form 2 is to be completed by the doctor treating the last illness, confirming the medical history, and attaching relevant extracts from the medical records. In a hospital setting, it could be the same person as that completing Form 1, but must be a senior doctor. In a community setting, the general practice with which the patient is registered has responsibility for completing the form. The Form 2 doctor has an option to express an opinion on the cause of death. Full coronial investigation is possible in either case, but is more likely when no expected cause of death is probable. This form is transmitted to the coroner's office.

Coronial certification is a process of analysis. The family of the deceased is consulted by a trained coronial investigator. Considering the information in Forms 1 and 2, the coroner can certify the death, after consultation with the deceased's family, or proceed to full coronial examination and inquiry. Random checks should be conducted on a portion of cases certified.

Expressing professional goals and duties is quite complex. Some are broad notions; others are more specific. There has been a move in recent times to simplify the ethical goals and duties for health care into broad principles, such as the following, espoused by American ethicists Beauchamp and Childress: beneficence, non-maleficence, autonomy, and justice. Beneficence encompasses the obligation to do good, to care for people, and non-maleficence is the paired obligation to do no harm to them. Autonomy is the principle of self-rule, of clients making decisions about their own lives. Justice is about fair distribution of resources, particularly when the pool of resources is limited.[18] British ethicist Gillon, proposes similar principles of respect for autonomy, beneficence, non-maleficence, and justice, but provides a slightly different definition of 'respect for autonomy', which he defines as 'the moral obligation to respect the autonomy of others in so far as such respect is compatible with equal respect for the autonomy of all potentially affected'.[19] In essence, this definition builds a social context into autonomy.

Slightly different principles have also been used to think about ethical duties, and proper behaviour, in health research practice. These research principles—beneficence, respect for persons, and justice—have, in the USA, been termed the Belmont principles because they were coined by the National Commission for the Protection of Human Subjects of Biomedical and Behavioural Research, in the Commission's Belmont Report. 'Beneficence', in the Commission's terms, concerns a dual obligation to, on the one hand, do no harm and promote the well-being of individuals, and on the other, to maximise potential benefit to society. 'Respect for persons' concerns an obligation to uphold the autonomy of individuals. The principle of justice concerns an obligation to share the benefits or burdens of research fairly in society.[20]

The principles suggested by Beauchamp and Childress (beneficence, non-maleficence, autonomy, and justice), and Gillon (respect for autonomy, beneficence, non-maleficence, and justice), and the Belmont principles (beneficence, respect for persons, and justice) have gained support because they provide a shorthand for thinking about ethics issues. The principles are used as tools to collect and summarise issues expressed by professionals, clients, and the community as being of concern. The principles are used as tools for ethical analysis and comparison. They do not, in themselves, give ultimate guidance on 'right' or 'wrong' behaviour.

The following dilemma is an exercise in using the principles to aid ethical reflection. The vignette is drawn from a study on ethics in the general practice setting in the mid 1990s: a group of multidisciplinary researchers and I asked general practitioners (GPs) and consumers of the services of GPs to nominate their ethics concerns. Vignettes were written to reflect these concerns, and the general practitioners and consumers were then convened to discuss possible solutions to the dilemmas contained in the vignettes.[21]

A 22-year-old man, Mr Y, had been very active until experiencing some unsettling symptoms. He saw his general practitioner, had a lot of tests, and eventually was diagnosed with early-stage multiple sclerosis. His GP said nothing much could be done at this stage, but advised Mr Y to stay active, and gave him something to help with that. The GP explained that this medication was called 'dexamethasone', and explained the dosage required, without giving further instructions. Mr Y was worried about the medication and was surprised to find out six months later, when he read the pharmacist's instructions, that he had been taking steroids.

In discussing the dilemma, many consumers focused on the responsibility they thought each patient should take to inform him or herself about the treatment being offered—this translates, in terms of the ethical principles discussed above, into the principle of autonomy. Consequently, they focused on the fact that Mr Y did not seek more information about the medication and did not read the pharmacy details until six months after purchasing the drug. The general practitioners however wondered at the apparent paternalism of the doctor, who had decided that acting beneficently did not include allowing the patient to make an informed decision.

The balance between possible long-term effects of steroids and the benefit in prescribing something to stave off early degeneration in multiple sclerosis could also be raised. If these steroids are thought to be beneficial, then under the principle of justice such drugs should be made equitably available to all those who might benefit. You could apply the same discussion to more recent drug treatments for multiple sclerosis. How then, should the care be delivered? There is a caution to be made here: justice is about the distribution of a good. This is different to the legal sense of justice. In other words, justice is a resource issue, as is explained further in Chapter 2. A further caution is that the autonomy at issue is the client's autonomy, not the professional's. Autonomy is discussed in some detail in Chapter 3. It is clear that, having summarised possible concerns, using the principles as an aid, further discussion needs to take place on the issues raised in the vignette. Neither the principles nor the summarising process alone solve the dilemma.

The Belmont principles—beneficence, respect for persons, and justice—were formulated to provide 'an analytical framework' to 'guide the resolutions of ethical problems' in research.[22] They may have been attractive to the Commission because of their practical application.[23] The principles represent a minimal position because they capture what is regarded as key issues in diverse ethics frameworks. Beauchamp and Childress also have stated that they came up with their principles of beneficence, non-maleficence, autonomy, and justice, despite their theoretical differences. Their theoretical positions are fundamentally different: Beauchamp's stance can be broadly described as utilitarian, whereas Childress's is, again generally speaking, deontological. A utilitarian concentrates on the outcome of behaviour for the greatest number, and aims for the happiness, or utility, of the greatest number in society. A deontologist, on the other hand, looks at the fundamental rule, or 'deon', that should be applied, in all situations, to ensure an ethical process. These theories are described further in Chapter 10. Beauchamp and Childress acknowledge that many different ethics theories can legitimately claim to have advanced health care ethics.[24]

The following two paragraphs discuss some of the support, advanced by different ethics theories and frameworks, for the principles of beneficence, non-maleficence, autonomy, and justice. The key idea is that each principle has its merits, even though different ethics theories and frameworks provide different supporting arguments. How much you emphasise each principle may shed some light on your overall ethical framework. This is discussed further in Chapter 3, in the section headed 'A dynamic relationship'. (You may decide to skip over the next two paragraphs now and return to them later when you feel ready to delve into ethics theory.)

Immanuel Kant was the founder of deontological theory. The central issue in Kant's deontological theory is the individual pursuit of morality. Freedom underpins Kant's theory, as it is needed for individuals to develop and act on their moral laws. A duty to uphold freedom entails respect for oneself, and respect for others. Although Kant rejects a perfect duty to benefit others and not to harm them, he maintains that a duty to benefit oneself and to refrain from harming oneself is part of the fundamental duty of respect. As respect for others is also fundamental, duties to benefit others and refrain from harming others stem from allowing them freedom to safeguard their own well-being. Justice implies that we fairly respect everyone's need to develop their own moral selves. It also implies the ultimate good of 'moral perfection'. The way of achieving moral perfection, according to Kant's theory, is to treat individuals with respect, and to extend that respect to all people equally, under a framework of justice as fairness. In other words, it stems from treating individuals with respect, and not as a means to an end.[25]

Utilitarian theory aims for the smallest possible amount of harm and the greatest possible amount of benefit. For utilitarians, beneficence involves maximising benefit and minimising harm. This is best achieved by allowing autonomy, because it is assumed that each person acts to pursue his or her own well-being and happiness. John Stuart Mill was a founder of utilitarianism. Under Mill's utilitarianism, liberty should be limited to a certain extent to allow for justice and the fair distribution of burden and benefit. Individual liberty is limited when exercising liberty may unreasonably infringe on others; liberty would be denied in circumstances in which other individuals were severely harmed or their similar liberties were threatened.[26]

The shorthand principles of beneficence, non-maleficence, autonomy, and justice make little sense on their own. They are simply tools, expressions of key ethical obligations that health care workers should fulfil, and goals to aim for. At best, the principles are a shorthand expression for drawing together concerns, and for referring to a considerable body of thought and literature about health care ethics. They extend the context for considering key issues in health care to the community and social contexts in which we live. At worst, the principles are used as a narrow and prescriptive decision-binding tool. It is not enough to think that summarising concerns under these, or similar, principles will lead to a solution. In addition to knowing the ethics principles, we have to constantly apply them within an ethical framework. We need to know our obligations, and we must live up to them.

In applying principles and meeting our obligations, the particular values and beliefs of the individuals and groups we care for, and the specific situations to which the principles are applied, must also be taken into account.[27] Professional standards, which reflect a shared sense of obligation, must be able to be communicated to relevant groups, and the ethics of relevant groups must be heard by professions. In essence, it is the issues themselves, not the umbrella, summarising principles, which should have prominence in ethical discussion and ethical analysis.

As simple, shorthand points, the principles of beneficence, non-maleficence, autonomy, and justice have the potential to be very useful. Many students and health professionals use them precisely because they are easily grasped, and applied. They do not, in themselves, provide answers for ethical dilemmas that you might face, but they do provide a starting place for reflection on ethics in your work as a health care worker. The lack of ready answers or solutions is perhaps a strength of the principles. The reality is that ethics is dynamic: times change; people change; medical problems and health issues change; and social contexts change. The principles will continue to be useful tools precisely because they do not lay down strict rules to be applied whatever the situation, culture, client, or professional involved.

In concise historical review of approaches to medical ethics, Edmund Pellegrino argues that some dissatisfaction with principles as they apply to specific cases has led us to a sceptical and chaotic chapter in ethics history. Yet, difficult decisions and clinical realities remain, so ethics reflection continues.[28]

This consideration of cases is how health care has been taught over generations. It is not incompatible at all with understanding important links and theories. In clinical case description, the story about an individual demonstrates 'what can happen' and serves as a guide on 'what to do'.[29] The teachers develop students' case-based reasoning and ensure students are exposed to enough diverse case situations that they have a broad and complex understanding of case management in clinical practice. This book is structured so that the focus is on the individual and their story. You are encouraged to think about ethics implications of health as each individual travels through the sequence of treatment with you. The stories you reflect on will challenge you ethically in the same way as your clinical reasoning is challenged as you develop it.

PROFESSIONAL GUIDELINES ON ETHICS

Individual reflection on standards, skill, and ethics is vital, yet individual reflection alone is problematic. It is difficult to act ethically without some guidance. Some of that guidance is found in discussion with fellow professionals, and some is found in written form, in professional codes of ethics. A profession is an occupation that:

- is skilled
- requires training to a high level (to which considerable time is devoted, which leads to the expectation of relatively high remuneration)
- gives rise to expectations of a high standard of proficiency
- is bound by a code of ethics of ideals of service to society.[30]

In professional life, there is some sense of setting moral rules and moral ideals. Moral rules may not be left to individual discretion as much as moral ideals. A moral rule is something that must be obeyed, and can therefore become a list of prohibitions, such as 'Thou shalt not kill'. In contrast, a moral ideal is something that should be strived for; it requires some positive action.[31] So, there is a sense that 'lower' limits of behaviour exist and that we should strive for 'upper' ideals. Since we should abide by moral rules, we would regard behaviour that breaks these rules with disfavour. We might be forgiving when ideals are not upheld, as long as the person strives for them in the future. A written code makes this more explicit, and provides members, as well as outsiders, with clear expectations of the rules and ideals that are central to the profession.

Ian Freckelton, a barrister with an interest in medical law and ethics, has also pointed to the partly 'aspirational' nature of professional codes of ethics. He asks what importance it may have if the aspirational aspects are broken. The important moral feature of professional codes of ethics may be the way they encourage striving for the aspirations.[32] While it may be difficult to sanction a professional for not achieving a high aspiration (a moral ideal), it may not be so difficult to sanction a professional who has broken a moral rule.

Philosophically, the principles that professions seek to uphold translate into moral rules that guide behaviour.[33] A sense of those rules is found in codes of ethics. Many different ethical frameworks support, to some extent, the notion of practical rules. But moral rules are especially important in rule forms of deontology and utilitarianism, which regard rules as ethically necessary.[34] Rules can be formed and adopted so that moral goals may be achieved. While the rules can be formed by individuals, according to Kant, the collective notion of shared rationality implies that rules formed by rational individuals will be shared and will have commonalities.[35] As a professional working in a community of other member professionals, you are expected to share some common 'professional ethics' rules, to have a sense of purpose in expressing those rules, and to strive to abide by them. Your strict professional duties can be defined with reference to the rules that your profession adopts. Your goals go further than that: you have a general duty to aspire to the optimal goals, to go, in other words, beyond minimum duties. Thus, goals and duties go hand in hand.

Codes of ethics can be thought of as 'general action guides' for professionals.[36] You, as a health care professional, are required to abide by your association's code of ethics in carrying out your work. Your code is a potential influence on your conduct, because it can define how you should act, and mould you to conform with your profession's standards. The code is a collective responsibility in the ethical conduct of health care by you and your fellow member professionals.[37] The codes may be evidence of existing ethics standards, rather than creating obligations in themselves. According to Knultgen, the purposes of professional codes are to promote a sense of community among members, to discipline the behaviour of members, and to ensure public trust in professional actions.[38] Knowledge of relevant standards is essential. Self-regulation of standards is formalised beyond complaints mechanisms in some jurisdictions. In Canada, physicians sit for re-registration exams every couple of years. As part of that, knowledge of clinical medicine and legal, ethical, and organisational aspects of medicine are tested. Standards of public interest obligations are the focus.[39]

Guidance on proper behaviour is crucial. As Hans Jonas has said, it is especially difficult to define ethical conduct in a technologically complex situation, as modern health care inevitably is. People who have relevant technological expertise can help to predict the consequences of actions. Without their help, actions, even if done with good intentions, could easily result in harm to others.[40]

This has particular relevance for health care teams that combine different sorts of expertise. You should get used to checking ethics limits with the whole team. The minimum is to check with your own peers. The importance of relying on others for guidance is evident even in Kant's otherwise individualist writings, which stress virtue in relation to one's own moral laws. According to Kant, the acceptability of actions to others is important because the praise of others is essential to reinforce virtuous actions.[41] In simple terms, you check and discuss matters with your colleagues to see if you have acted properly or if your planned action is ethical. It seems appropriate that the group of people who best understand the professional skill and actions involved are ethically active, in effect setting their own goals and limits. We become worried if outsiders have too much control over the ethics of a profession. As one commentator has stated, 'a morality of those whose hands are clean only because they have the position of an observer, charging others with the responsibility, seems doubtful'.[42]

But if professions fail to set their standards, and outsiders are worried about standards, outsiders may well step in and set the limits of acceptable professional conduct. Professions have sometimes refined and discussed their standards precisely because of the threat of such external imposition of standards. They should be wary of thinking that the community trusts them entirely. Distrust of professions on the part of the general public has been reported in the early 1990s. The public fears that professionals enter into their chosen field solely, or primarily, to gain money and prestige; and that professionals are held captive by business interests rather than being bound by the traditional values of service.[43] Sociological concerns about the integrity of professionals include the arguments that professional ethics:

* is a product of powerful institutions, and
* is merely a tool of monopolisation, such that the 'values' of any profession are constructed to serve the interests of the profession, and group ethics is imperfectly internalised, and ultimately, is neither shared nor acted on by individual professionals.[44]

If this distrust continues, society may judge that more outside regulation is needed, effectively limiting the power and discretion of professionals. The community trust in professional standards is premised on the expectation that the community as a whole will ultimately be served by the profession.

Professional codes of ethics continue to have prominence because they do provide some guidance, even if that guidance is not complete and is employed differently by different individuals. Internal regulation and standard setting can also be used constructively. Continual assessment of the existing standards in the codes of ethics is needed as part of ethical reflection. The formation of the code is itself a valuable ethical process, and as is explained by business ethicists Stephen Cohen and Damian Grace, the process of reflection is perhaps ethically more important than enshrining a code.[45] However, the process of forming an ethical code should not replace individual conscience and reflection; we need to distinguish between teaching of custom (or group norms) and what is moral.[46]

Exercise 1.4 General principles in your professional code of ethics

You should have at hand your professional code of ethics. If you do not already have it, you could try looking up the association website, ringing your association to have one mailed to you, or visiting a library where it may be held. Examples of the latest codes of ethics for nurses and doctors can be found on association websites, such as those of the Australian Medical Association (updated in 2003, at <www.ama.com.au>), the Australian Nursing Council (updated in 2002, at <www.anci.org.au>), or the New Zealand Medical Association (updated in 2002, at <www.nzma.org.nz>). These outline duties to patients, the community, and the profession. You should remember to obtain updates whenever your code is altered.

Using your own code, try the following exercise. Fill in the grid provided for you, placing the principles and comments of guidance in your code of ethics under the broad headings of beneficence, non-maleficence, autonomy, and justice. You may like to refresh your memory on the definition of these principles, according to Beauchamp and Childress. The definitions were provided for you earlier in this chapter. If you want to concentrate on research ethics, you may wish to alter the headings to those of the Belmont principles: beneficence, respect for persons, and justice.

Code of ethics

My profession is:

....

....

....

Principles of note in my code of ethics

BENEFICENCE

....

....

....

....

....

....

NON-MALEFICENCE

....

....

....

....

....

....

AUTONOMY

....

....

....

....

....

....

JUSTICE

....

....

....

....

....

....

There is an existing body of research on professional codes of ethics. An overview of codes and declarations of ethics has been undertaken by Raanon Gillon.[47] The oaths that medical students swear to abide by have also been examined, and have been found to be less than comprehensive in the way they deal with the principles of beneficence, non-maleficence, autonomy, and justice. They were found to be particularly scant in relation to the principle of autonomy.[48] In an early study comparing professional codes of research ethics, a co-investigator and I found that codes of ethics of Australian health professions on research practice differed in what issues and obligations they emphasised. Some seemed to value autonomy more than others, and few explicitly considered justice.[49] Nursing codes and medical codes are frequently compared, and it has been noted that they differ in their emphasis on autonomy.[50] Nowadays, the concept of autonomy is frequently balanced by concerns of resource availability for all, and limits of professional responsibilities.

Codes need to provide some detailed guidance. General principles alone are not sufficient. Australia's own National Health and Medical Research Council (NHMRC) is particularly aware of this, and seeks to respond to significant advances in medical research by holding forums and producing discussion documents in addition to the *National Statement on Ethical Conduct in Research Involving Humans*, the principles for research conduct. A separate manual has been produced to guide researchers and ethics committees in their deliberations.[51] More on research is included in Chapter 9.

Having a code of ethics is, in itself, not sufficient. Codes of ethics need to be more than window dressing, and there is a strong potential for criticism if they are thought to be either rarely enforced or rarely applied by practitioners.[52] At the heart of the potential criticism is that, having established professional codes of ethics, and justified them if need be, professionals also need some mechanism for giving effect to those ethics, beyond that of the virtue of the individual health care worker. More on mechanisms which give effect to codes and standards of behaviour is included in Chapter 8.

From time to time, guidelines are updated. Examining the historical development of codes is also an interesting exercise. As a profession develops, and the context in which it is called to practise changes, so codes become increasingly defined. Research guidelines and codes are a good example of this. Different professions applying their own particular codes of ethics can make different assessments of the same situation. You must be ready to be part of discussion and to be alert to changes in context and professional bounds.

To follow group-defined ethics standards, without making an input into the evolving standards, would be a minimal position to take. It is preferable that all professional members actively consider their ethical stance and be ready to explain it or pursue further discussion on it. Opportunities for discussion and explanation often arise on a casual basis; for example, in the tea room, at handover, at professional conferences over lunch, or as you talk about what happened during the day with your flatmates or partner. Professional discussions can also be scheduled if there is an issue that seems to be arising consistently or is of some moment. These meetings and discussions are of utmost importance to the dynamic nature of health care ethics.

The philosopher John Rawls thought that principles of conduct, such as we find in some codes of ethics, were important. He also thought that we need more than principles to bring ethics into action. Rawls distinguished between the principles and the subsequent judgements of value in relation to those principles.[53] We need to make individual, and collective, judgements before principles are put into practice.

Think about one of the basic principles that you might find in your code of ethics (some website suggestions for association codes were noted above—you might like to make use of one of them, instead of your own). Think of situations in which you have applied this principle and make a note of how you have seen others apply it.

You may apply it slightly differently to another health care worker, or someone else in your own profession. Part of that difference may be the values that you use when you interpret and apply the principle. One of Rawls's points is that the judgements we make may depend on the contractual situation to which principles and values are applied (the word 'contractual' here is being used to refer to any agreement, whether implied or explicit, between people). We can expect some differences in 'ethical behaviour'. Just because someone behaves differently does not necessarily mean that they are unethical. It does give us pause for reflection and discussion though. The next time you see something quite different in application of a principle, take a moment to think about the values that may have influenced that professional's behaviour, and the contractual situation in which it was applied. You may be witness to extreme values or a contractual situation that puts considerable constraints on professional behaviour. One type of constraint, the social and institutional constraint, is explored further in Chapter 7.

An editorial written by the former Director-General of the World Health Organization (WHO), Dr Hiroshi Nakajima, reinforced the need for, and the value of, professional expressions of ethics in professional codes.[54] Some profession-driven defining and expression of ethics aims and objectives is, in part, what forms a profession and guides members' good practice. However, Dr Nakajima also highlighted the importance of community discussion and debate on ethics. Health care is, after all, professional caring in context. He emphasised the diversity of values in the community, which should be borne in mind as professionals begin their task of offering health care.

> To be ethical, our responses must be both honest and humane: first, they must be applicable to people's concrete circumstances, and meaningful to them; and second, they must be respectful of their rights, values and personal dilemmas, as lived within their own communities. In other words, ethical issues must be worked out with the people concerned.
>
> Values cannot be imposed from the outside, but a very active search is needed for convergence in the values which guide our health work and policies. To foster health development and international health action in a spirit of respect, solidarity and equity, WHO's first responsibility must be to promote a genuinely open dialogue involving all peoples, cultures and health-related groups and institutions. All partners concerned, both within and outside the Organization, should feel authorized to speak and be heard with respect and attention.[55]

More on community input is included in Chapter 7. The issue of individual client input is discussed throughout this book.

CARING IN MULTIDISCIPLINARY TEAMS

We live and work in the reality of different professions in health care. Different professions train their members in different skills, and these differently skilled workers all tackle health care together. The basic aim of all health professions is to care for clients or patients, to be beneficent towards them and the community that is served. Yet sometimes, there seems to be differences in attitude among health professionals. You may seem to be at loggerheads over health-system priorities, or decisions over individual client care. Despite your differences, you must learn to work together, because you need each other's skills to provide proper health care.

One step towards working well together is to understand each other's different skills and different objectives in providing care. A common example of two professions working together is that of doctors and nurses. Nurses acknowledge both the difficulty and the importance of working together with doctors, who have different skills and objectives. Working as a team does not mean always working 'under' another profession. It means being aware of and working towards goals, and on occasions being 'guided by others who possess greater knowledge and expertise'.[56] Of course, establishing team leadership will depend on the goals aimed for and who has the skills to lead the team towards that goal. Junior residents find themselves learning a great deal from senior charge nurses. Experienced nurses and their favourite doctors appear to work effortlessly. Perhaps they have come to a common understanding of the goals of care in their own context and appreciate each other's skills so much that there is true team harmony in providing that care. You could apply the same assessment of successful teamwork in other professional combinations.

Discussing basic values and objectives in health care with the multidisciplinary teams with which you work can be useful in establishing a common ground and acceptable aims. There are philosophical processes that can help us to achieve this, such as those that rely on relativism and understanding of different cultural stances and beliefs. Yet, there is also a danger, as noted by Moreno, that aiming for consensus too early, and sacrificing differences of opinion to achieve that consensus, can hide the difficulty of an issue, or can even hide divergent views on an issue.[57]

Harman is a philosopher who has defended relativism, a theory that suggests that there are no hard and fast rules in ethics. Rather, ethics can change depending on the perspectives of key participants in a dilemma, and depending on the stance of the group to which they belong. Not all people agree with relativism. It is useful to think about here though, because it stresses how an agreement can be reached between people with different perspectives on what might be best or right. Harman claims that a judgement of proper conduct by one party towards another depends on the agreement between the two parties.[58] In a practitioner–client relationship, both parties should agree that what is being undertaken is proper. In the context of a health care team, the team should also agree that it is proper. Reaching this agreement does not necessarily mean minimal standards. In any contractual situation, an upper level, beyond a bare minimum, can be negotiated. The discussion in this book is based on the assumption that an optimal level of ethics behaviour is what should be sought—that is, it assumes that we should strive to go beyond the minimum and aim for an outcome that will raise and uphold standards.

When tasks and responsibilities are divided in a health care team, it is easy to lose sight of the fact that the team, as a whole, is responsible for the care of the individual patient. You routinely work in teams that share skills and responsibility for client care. When you are part of that system, the standards of care from each of the health care professions apply. Everyone would do well to acknowledge a team ethic of caring. It is worth spending time with one's own team, discussing and defining team goals, and minimum rules and optimal ideals, so that compatibilities are recognised, and potential problem areas are identified before they occur in practice. In an interdisciplinary approach to ethics education at a US University Health Center, one benefit was thought to be a complexity of issues that different training professionals brought to the ethics discussion. The lecturers felt that when students understood each of the team members' roles and responsibilities, they had the prerequisite for then discharging their ethical obligations to their patients.[59] So, the ethics discussion and decision cannot be in isolation from other members for it to be realistic. The development of both professional team responsibility and team ethics that are specific to our work practices is a valuable and practical addition to our implementation of professional ethics. In the future, the concepts of team responsibility and team ethics may also pose a challenge to those reforming law and regulatory mechanisms. At the moment, legal doctrines and frameworks do not deal with the concept of team responsibility as well as the non-legal concept of one's professional responsibility to one's client.[60] This is most apparent when legal redress is sought in health care situations; in negligence actions, for instance.

Knowledge of the ethics stances of both parties is vital in arriving at an agreed standard of behaviour in multidisciplinary teams. Each party needs to express their expectations of appropriate conduct. Think about where you can find up-to-date versions of different stances of professionals that you are likely to work with, and keep a note for yourself to stay in touch with updates from time to time. Also, think about opportunities for your team to talk about ethics concerns and expectations.

As in any process of social negotiation, agreement on ethical conduct may change. Appropriate standards are, therefore, dynamic rather than static, fluid rather than absolute. They may be different in different situations and at different times. This book highlights what would be acceptable as you, the health care professional, begin to work in health care and in treatment relationships with clients—acceptable to the professions, the clients, and the community.

Summary of key issues

- Fundamental values
- Debate and reflection
- Skill and limits
- Caring and commitment
- Goals and duties
- Codes of practice
- Principles: beneficence, non-maleficence, autonomy, and justice
- Judging the importance of principles, and applying principles

Notes

1   D. Collinson, *Fifty Major Philosophers: A Reference Guide*, Routledge, London, 1987, p. 16.
2   T. L. Beauchamp and J. F. Childress, *Principles of Biomedical Ethics*, 4th edn, Oxford University Press, London, 1994, p. 465.
3   Collinson, p. 21.
4   S. F. Spicker, I. Alon, A. de Vries, and H. T. Engelhardt Jr, *The Use of Human Beings in Research,* Philosophy and Medicine 28, Kluwer Academic Publishers, Dordrecht, 1988.
5   C. A. Berglund, K. Mitchell, and K. Cox, *Exploring Clinical Ethics*, 2nd edn, distance-education module in a Masters of Clinical Education course, University of New South Wales, 1993, p. 4.
6   E. D. Pellegrino, 'Character, Virtue and Self-interest in the Ethics of the Professions', *Journal of Contemporary Health Law and Policy*, vol. 5, 1989, p. 56.
7   See, for example, E. M. Hubert, D. Douglas-Stelle, and J. Bickel, 'Context in Medical Education: the Informal Ethics Curriculum', *Medical Education*, vol. 30, 1996, pp. 353–64.
8   S. F. Barker, 'What is a Profession?', *Professional Ethics: A Multidisciplinary Journal*, vol. 1, nos. 1&2, 1992, p. 86.
9   T. L. Beauchamp and J. F. Childress, *Principles of Biomedical Ethics*, 5th edn, Oxford University Press, New York, 2001, p. 45.
10 K. Marino, *Resumes for the Health Care Professional*, John Wiley & Sons, New York, 1993, p. 36.
11 Marino, pp. 37, 39.
12 'Hospital Faker Ends in Doc', *Sydney Morning Herald* (reprinted from Reuters), 30 December 1995, p. 10.
13 'Doctor Helped Woman Commit Suicide', *Sydney Morning Herald* (reproduced from the *New York Times*), 7 June 1990, p. 12.
14 J. Smith, 'The Shipman Inquiry. Third Report: Death Certification and Investigation of Deaths by Coroners.' Presented to Parliament by the Secretary of State for the Home Department and the Secretary of State for Health by Command of Her Majesty July 2003. Cm5854. Whitehall, London, July 2003.
15 S. Ramsay, 'Audit further exposes UK's worst serial killer', [news] *The Lancet*, vol. 357, 2001, pp. 123–5.
16 R. Horton, 'The real lessons from Harold Frederick Shipman', *The Lancet*, vol. 357, 2001, pp. 82–3.
17 Smith, The Shipman Inquiry, Third Report.
18 T. L. Beauchamp and J. F. Childress, *Principles of Biomedical Ethics*, 4th edn, Oxford University Press, New York, 1994, p. 38.
19 R. Gillon, 'Introduction', in R. Gillon (ed.), *Principles of Health Care Ethics*, John Wiley & Sons, Chichester, 1994, p. xxii.
20 United States Department of Health, Education, and Welfare. *Ethical Principles and Guidelines for the Protection of Human Subjects of Research* [The Belmont Report], publication no. OS 78–0012, United States Department of Health, Education, and Welfare, Washington DC, 1978, pp. 4–10.
21 C. A. Berglund, C. D. Pond, M. F. Harris, P. M. McNeill, D. Gietzelt, E. Comino, V. Traynor, E. Meldrum, and C. Boland, 'The Formation of Professional and Consumer Solutions: Ethics in the General Practice Setting', *Health Care Analysis*, vol. 5, no. 2, 1997, pp. 164–7.

22 The Belmont Report, p. 2.

23 D. De Grazia, 'Moving Forward in Bioethical Theory: Theories, Cases, and Specified Principlism', *Journal of Medicine and Philosophy*, vol. 17, 1992, p. 515.

24 Beauchamp and Childress, p. 45.

25 R. J. Sullivan, *Immanuel Kant's Moral Theory*, Cambridge University Press, Cambridge, 1989, pp. 46, 104, 105, 203, 207, 208, 234.

26 J. S. Mill, 'On Liberty', in *Three Essays*, Oxford University Press, London, 1975, pp. 94, 96.

27 B. A. Lustig, 'The Method of "Principlism": A Critique of the Critique', *Journal of Medicine and Philosophy*, vol. 17, 1992, p. 498.

28 E. Pellegrino, 'The metamorphosis of medical ethics: A 30 year retrospective', *Journal of the American Medical Association*, vol. 269, no. 9, 1993, pp. 1158–62.

29 K. Cox, 'Stories as case knowledge: case knowledge as stories', *Medical Education*, vol. 35, 2001, pp. 862–6.

30 Barker, pp. 73–99. See also Appendices 1, 2, and 3, in this book.

31 B. Gert, 'Morality, Moral Theory, and Applied and Professional Ethics', *Professional Ethics: A Multidisciplinary Journal*, vol. 1, nos 1&2, 1992, p. 19.

32 I. Freckelton, 'Enforcement of Ethics', in M. Coady and S. Bloch (eds), *Codes of Ethics and the Professions*, Melbourne University Press, Melbourne, 1996, p. 134.

33 W. D. Solomon, 'Rules and Principles', in W. T. Reich (ed.), *Encyclopedia of Bioethics*, vol. 1, The Free Press, New York, 1978, p. 410.

34 For a discussion of utilitarianism and deontology, see Beauchamp and Childress, p. 45.

35 Sullivan, p. 214.

36 Solomon, p. 407.

37 T. Tomaszewski, 'Ethical Issues from an International Perspective', *International Journal of Psychology*, vol. 124, 1979, p. 31.

38 J. Knultgen, *Ethics and Professionalism*, University of Pennsylvania Press, Philadelphia, 1988, pp. 212, 213, 215.

39 Medical Council of Canada. 'CLEO: Objectives of the Considerations of the Legal, Ethical and Organizational Aspects of the Practice of Medicine.' Medical Council of Canada, Ottawa, Ontario, 1999.

40 H. Jonas, *The Imperative of Responsibility: In Search of an Ethics for the Technological Age*, University of Chicago Press, Chicago, 1984, pp. 5–6.

41 Sullivan, p. 29.

42 Tomaszewski, pp. 131–5.

43 B. McDowell, 'The Excuses that Make Professional Ethics Irrelevant', *Professional Ethics: A Multidisciplinary Journal*, vol. 3, nos 3&4, 1994, p. 157.

44 J. L. Berlant, *Profession and Monopoly: A Study of Medicine in the United States and Great Britain*, University of California Press, Berkeley, 1975, pp. 29, 48, 55, 64.

45 A-M. Moodie, 'A Code of Ethics Doesn't Ensure Business Ethics', *Australian Financial Review*, 18 July 1997, p. 61, quoted in S. Cohen and D. Grace, *Business Ethics*, Oxford University Press, Melbourne, 1995.

46 See the discussion of the work of Joseph Butler in Collinson, p. 79.

47 R. Gillon, 'Medical Oaths, Declarations, and Codes', *British Medical Journal*, vol. 290, 1985, pp. 1194–5.

48 E. Dickenstein, J. Erlen, and J. A. Erlen, 'Ethical Principles Contained in Currently Professed Medical Oaths', *Academic Medicine*, vol. 66, no. 10, 1991, pp. 622–4.

49 C. A. Berglund and P. M. McNeill, 'Guidelines for Research Practice in Australia: NHMRC Statement & Professional Codes', *Community Health Studies*, vol. 13, no. 2, 1989, pp. 121–9.

50 M-J. Johnstone, 'Bioethics and the Wider Community: A Nursing Perspective', in *Proceedings of the First Annual Bioethics Association Conference: Bioethics and the Wider Community*, Bioethics Association, University of Melbourne, 5–7 April, 1991, pp. 103–16.

51 National Health and Medical Research Council, *National Statement on Ethical Conduct in Research Involving Humans*, Canberra, AGPS, 1999; and National Health and Medical Research Council, *Human Research Ethics Handbook: Commentary on the National Statement on Ethical Conduct in Research Involving Humans*, endorsed 25 October 2001, Canberra, AGPS, 2002.

52 B. Malley, 'Professionalism and Professional Ethics', in D. E. Edgar (ed.), *Social Change in Australia*, Cheshire, Melbourne, 1974, pp. 407–8.

53 J. A. Rawls, *A Theory of Justice*, Belknap Press, Harvard, 1971, pp. 20, 48, 120, 579.

54 H. Nakajima, 'Health, Ethics and Human Rights', *World Health*, 49th year, no. 5, September–October, 1996, p. 3.

55 Nakajima, p. 3.

56 A. Alexandra and A. Woodruff, 'A Code of Ethics for the Nursing Profession', in M. Coady and S. Bloch (eds), *Codes of Ethics and the Professions*, Melbourne University Press, Melbourne, 1996, p. 242.

57 J. D. Moreno, *Deciding Together: Bioethics and Moral Consensus*, Oxford University Press, New York, 1995.

58 G. Harman, 'Moral Relativism Defended', *Philosophical Review*, vol. 84, 1975, p. 3.

59 M. Yarborough, T. Jones, T. A. Cyr, S. Phillips, and D. Stelzner, 'Interprofessional education in ethics at an academic health sciences center', *Academic Medicine*, vol. 75, no. 8, 2000, pp. 793–800, at p. 794.

60 J. Hamblin, 'Let's Make it Legal: Morality and the Law', paper delivered at a meeting on equity and rationing in health care, at the Centre for Values, Ethics and the Law in Medicine, Sydney University, 11 November 1996.

2

Caring as service provision

Overview

- Accepting a job to provide service
- The business of provision
- Pharmaceuticals and the development of new drugs
- Patients/clients as consumers

The second chapter focuses on professional caring in terms of service availability. Justice issues are the focus. Models of justice are discussed, and examples of different models in action are worked through, both in terms of availability and access. Case studies are provided of treatments that are commonly available and those that are not. The development of drugs is also used as a case study.

ACCEPTING A JOB TO PROVIDE SERVICE

When you are applying for a job, you should consider the values of the institution, and the aims it pursues; in other words, the way the institutional services are delivered. The values and objectives of health care institutions differ. Even though they all aim to provide goods and deliver health care, how they define goods, and how they deliver health care can vary subtly. Sometimes this is because of the underlying ethic or morality system of the institution, such as in Catholic hospitals, and in Seventh Day Adventist hospitals. If you work in an institution, it is worth taking the time to find out what its values and objectives are. These values and objectives comprise more than just what sort of services the unit aims to provide, which is more easily discovered.[1] You may be able to discover from such statistical summary documents as Year Books that the hospital offers day surgery and specialises in skin treatments, or in fertility treatments. What is offered is only part of the information that you need.

Make a note of the goals or mission statement of a hospital near you, and of your own prospective or current place of employment. Once you find out the values, you need to decide whether that objective and the way it is achieved is compatible with your ethics and belief system.

Employees are part of the team that goes about distributing health resources. At some point, it would be useful to reflect on the model of distribution that is applied where you work. Taking time to think about how the organisation is set up will inform your reflection on any difficulties you face in securing resources, or in making your idea of a health service a reality for your clients.

The way resources are distributed is a 'justice' concern. You will remember that this was touched on in Chapter 1, in the discussion on definitions of the principles of beneficence, non-maleficence, autonomy (or 'respect for persons'), and justice. The idea of justice has many underlying assumptions. Generally speaking, it is about the fair distribution of burden and benefit. How you think about justice depends on your values and what you think health care should achieve.

Exercise 2.1 The sharing of resources

Take a moment to answer the following questions in the space below: What is the good that you think health care should aim for? How do you think that good should be shared around?

Your answer to the first question will depend on a value judgement of what is a good. Your answer to the second question will depend on whether you think people have a right to receive that good. Bear in mind that the word 'good' is used as a noun here, it is generally speaking a thing or concept when we talk about justice, not an adjective.

Many people would write something like 'health' or 'life' or 'quality of life' or 'health care' or 'treatment' in answer to the first question. Value judgements such as 'when needed' or 'when available' or 'when reasonable' or 'shared equally' are frequent responses to the second question. Thinking about how the way services are delivered shows us what sort of distribution is in action. If your health care institution has a queue system, or waiting times before a booking can be made, some ordering of patients is happening behind the scenes, before you, as a health practitioner, even see them.

If you wrote 'when affordable' or 'when reasonable' in answer to the second question you are assuming that there are competing claims on health resources. Competing claims on the system is the reality of modern health care. Before we can decide what is reasonable, we may need to know how large the pool of resources is, including the source of the money that fuels the system, and what and who else requires resources from the pool. The question of who decides on how to prioritise resources (should it be a clinician or someone who doesn't deal directly with clients?) is also a crucial justice question.

Your own idea of when you are available to work makes a difference to the type of work that you will do as well. Is 2 a.m. within your idea of proper availability of services? If it is, do you work that shift because your view is that that service should be available? Examining your own individual commitment to the type and availability of services that will be provided becomes part of the system. A system is, after all, made up of many people like you who have chosen to become health care professionals. Ethics can help with these difficult questions, by examining the good that is aimed for and the models of justice that guide the distribution of that good.

Doing good is the basic premise of being beneficent, of caring. To 'do good' requires understanding what 'good' is, and then acting to the extent of your responsibility to that good. It is an active obligation. Each profession has its own definition of 'a good' (the word 'good' here is being used in the general sense of 'aiming for good' and avoiding harm; it is not restricted to 'good' used as a noun—for example, delivering a 'good', where 'good' means health care services). For example, to an obstetrician or midwife, it may be the preservation of life; to a palliative care specialist, it may be an 'easy death'; while to a rehabilitation team, it may be 'quality of life'. Getting consensus on what a good is (within a profession, or group of professions in the one system) is the first step in deciding reasonable beneficence responsibilities. Since that good must then be distributed this consensus is also important in deciding justice responsibilities. The arrived at definition is an ideal, so while the good might not be achieved all the time, the ethical position is to continue to aim for it, thereby maximising the possibility of doing good and minimising the possibility of doing harm.

You may take the view that the profession should not define what a good is at all, and that nobody can really define the good to aim for except the client. If you take that view, you would be an extreme libertarian. As J. S. Mill, the most quoted libertarian, writes, each person can and should decide for themselves what is in their best interest; having decided what is in their best interest, that person has a right to it, unless it conflicts with similar rights of others, or threatens the fabric of society.[2] This position places autonomy first, unless it can be argued, under fairly limited circumstances, that autonomy cannot be granted. The extreme libertarian position would place client choice first, rather than the current or available professional view of what is the best treatment. Whether or not autonomy and the client's wish, or choice, should override the professional's view of beneficence (what they think is reasonable care, or the best care to provide), is discussed further in Chapter 3.

However, most health care systems, by definition, do not only respond to what each individual wants. They try to decide what is a good, thereby anticipating what people will want and need, and make resource allocation decisions on that basis. Most systems are, therefore, not strictly libertarian. However, the limits that Mill identifies as reasonable limits to autonomy are useful in that they may well reflect rights that we are prepared to acknowledge within an existing health care system.

You may decide that acting beneficently is only required when someone has a right to whatever good you would be promoting. You would be correct because there is a difference between rights and interests. That can be illustrated fairly easily, with an exercise that works best in a group. First, ask 'Who owns a car?' Many hands will probably go up. The rest of the group may have an interest in those cars, but they don't necessarily have a right to them ... or do they? The people with the goods (the cars) might be caring for others by giving their cars to people without them, but is that an obligation? Ask the people with the cars: 'Who would give their car to someone who doesn't have one?' Wait, and watch the hands disappear. So, what interests are reasonable? Perhaps if I told you that I want your car so that I can get to work more easily, or so I can get to university to study, you might feel swayed. Can I have it? I have shown you a good reason why I want it. I have asked, and made my autonomous decision clear. Do you have a duty to give the car to me?

Under our current societal structure, the answer to this question is 'probably not', and the same applies to whatever else I ask for, unless there is model of justice operating that obliges you to fulfil that wish or want. You will see more on wishes and autonomy in Chapter 3. If I was to take your car, I might be depriving your similar interest to get to work or to university. There is also the consideration that you have probably earned the car by buying it. All is not lost though. Society does acknowledge my interest in coming to work, or university, and makes public transport available at a reasonable cost. There are some human-rights agreements, for example the United Nations International Covenant on

Civil and Political Rights, that regard education as a basic right, but only to the level of a decent minimum.[3] Studying or working is seen as a good, so my interest in pursuing that is reasonable, but getting there quickly or more conveniently may not be pursued to the exclusion of others' interests. There is a similar limit to beneficence obligations in health care. Like access to education, it is thought that we only have a right to certain levels of beneficence; beyond those levels our right becomes an interest only.

The two-tiered nature of the Australian health care system reflects this division of health care into 'rights' and 'interests'. There is a publicly funded, government-provided sector and a privately funded, privately provided sector. While these are designed to operate in parallel, there is constant debate about what should be publicly available, and how much public provision should be available to those who can afford private care.[4] More detail on our health system is included under the next subheading in this chapter, 'The business of provision'. Medicare provides automatic cover for many aspects of basic, or decent, minimum health care but not for 'extras' like private rooms in hospital or patient choice of doctor. Patients who are not privately covered must pay for extras somehow. Thus, we could say that the minimum covered under Medicare is considered a right, while the public is only thought to have an interest in the extras for which they must pay.

Another example of the distinction between rights and interests is advice on diet to prevent heart disease. Such advice is a good that is so fundamental to health that it is currently seen as a right—publicly funded dietary advice begins in early childhood clinics and at primary school. In contrast transplant of a diseased heart is not seen as a right; we know this because this treatment option is not made available to all. Looking into the future, a life-saving heart transplant may one day be seen as a 'right' (given sufficient hearts available), but repeated heart transplants may not. Medical treatment after life-threatening injury is, under our current system, a near absolute right because life itself is threatened, and our concept of a right to health holds our right to life fundamental. However, we may not have such an absolute right to receive counselling after injury, because although it could be argued to be essential to recovering a decent minimum of health, it may not be available in places that are convenient to the client, or at hours that suit them perfectly. It may even be left to state or regional bodies to decide how much of a right or interest counselling is.

As a general rule of thumb, when there is strong agreement that service obligations are mandated, that service will be a right. When there appears to be considerable discretion about whether or not to provide the service, the service is meeting a strong interest (or claim), not a right.

Raanon Gillon has noted the difference between institutional and moral rights: institutional rights are simply claims that have been justified. The institution can decide, collectively, to grant such things as free medical care, but equally, it may take those things away. Moral rights, on the other hand, cannot be taken away. Gillon also notes that only some rights impose obligations on others to act in a particular way.[5] This distinction between rights that impose obligations and those that don't is not new to the law field, which tries to clarify which of our obligations are contractual, and therefore enforceable, and which are merely good-will. Jurist and theorist, W. N. Hohfeld, outlined the difference between wishes, or liberties, and 'claim-rights'. The latter imply an obligation on others to satisfy those claims. The former do not.[6] Daniel Callahan, an eminent ethicist from the USA, also notes that there are limits to our ability to satisfy health interests. He argues that before we talk in terms of health rights, we must re-examine the fundamental goals of medicine (paying particular attention to how realistic and affordable those goals are) and countries must meet agreed–upon goals.[7]

Applying the concept of good, whether it is an absolute or decent minimum, is an illustration of the breadth of responsibilities to do good that health care professionals undertake. Many codes of ethics mention acting in the patient's or client's best interests, and furthering the health of the community. A professional's responsibility is not only to treat each client, but also to ensure that others have the opportunity to be similarly treated. In other words, the individual treatment that a professional gives to his or her client should not compromise the availability of such treatment to others. In simple terms, questions of individual client care, and doing good for them, come under the concept or principle of beneficence. The community obligation that is part of beneficence is also related to the principle of justice, in that it is about questions of the distribution of, and access to, health care.

By now you will have realised that accepting a job to be a health care worker, and providing care, has a professional, community, institutional, and societal context. If you are to remain responsible by world standards, you may need to check, every now and then, that how you approach the business of providing is consistent with the expectations that are expressed in international documents on human rights. Those expectations can appear to be quite stringent. WHO has defined health as 'a state of complete physical, mental, and social wellbeing and not merely the absence of disease or infirmity'. WHO's health goal for your clients and potential clients, which is essentially the good we should all be striving for, is expressed in the preamble to the constitution of WHO: 'The enjoyment of the highest attainable standard of health is one of the fundamental rights of every human being without distinction of race, religion, political belief, economic or social condition'. These objectives were viewed as ambitious at the start of the new century but are used as a guiding mandate to tackle such issues as preventable transmission of HIV, and attainable improvements in basic living conditions and health care access for all people.[8]

All health care workers struggle to provide 'a good', however they define it, in a context of competing claims on resources, and seemingly diminishing pools of those resources.

There are a number of philosophical choices to be made, under the principle of justice, in deciding just how to distribute what is available. In Australia, the pool of resources for health care is limited to 8.5 per cent of gross domestic product (GDP). This is high compared with some countries in the OECD (Organization for Economic Cooperation and Development), but low compared with the USA, in which an estimated 13.9 per cent of GDP is spent on health care.[9] (Some would argue that there is great inequity in the United States system, despite the larger GDP available, and there is a constant review, in the USA, of how to better distribute care.) The proportion of funds available for health care is unlikely to change quickly. So the question is, given the current pool of resources, how can we distribute what we have in an ethical manner?

Three models of justice

The three justice models discussed most often are: justice as fairness, comparative justice, and distributive justice. They derive from the philosophical writings of three well-known philosophers, and as the discussion progresses, you will notice that each model has different ethical theories or frameworks supporting it. All these theories and frameworks are about what a society might regard as fair distribution of limited resources that are in demand by the members of the society.

The philosopher John Rawls writes about the concept of justice as fairness. It is a concept of absolute equality and fairness. The model has been applied, by others, to health, and is the justice model that is closest to the WHO definition of health.[10] Disparate treatment based on the financial circumstances, race, or any number of other distinguishing features of those to whom services are being provided, is unacceptable under the justice-as-fairness model. The justice-as-fairness model cuts across lines created by nations or regions: nationality or place of residence do not determine rights to health care. Under this model of justice, differential treatment is justified only to compensate for disadvantages suffered by some people. The aim is that all people should end up roughly equal.

Think about what limits your clients in achieving health. Should the removal of barriers to health be part of the health care agenda?

Aboriginal education models are now incorporating culture and community into a holistic approach to health. This is only one example of services that aim to alleviate historically accrued disadvantages and barriers as well as putting in place physical health measures in the pursuit of health.

Comparative justice, as its name suggests, involves assessing the relative importance of people's interests in receiving the health resource. The philosopher David Hume was primarily concerned with comparative justice and with acknowledging the limited nature of resources. His model of comparative justice is a compromise between justice as fairness, in which the ideal is providing treatment based on nothing else but need, and acknowledging the limited pool of resources from which to provide that treatment. The triage system of health care delivery is an example of the comparative justice model in action: need assessment is carried out and treatment is given accordingly. Minor complaints wait longer, and more serious cases are rushed to the top of the queue.

A type of triage system exists in our emergency/casualty departments. It also exists in our waiting lists for public hospital care. The following extract from the New South Wales Department of Health policy guidelines on prioritising patients on elective waiting lists is an example of the assessment of need that is the key to the triage system. Emergency admissions are excluded from this, as they are assumed to take place immediately.

What do you think about the following, as quoted from the policy guideline?

The Department is committed to improving the way in which hospital booking lists are managed across the public hospital system and to ensure that patients receive access to health care on the basis of clinical need and not as a result of other factors such as their health insurance status.

The priority is in three main categories:

Category 1—Urgent
Admission within seven days is required for a serious condition or one causing a high level of pain, severe disability or having the potential to deteriorate quickly to the point that it may become an emergency.

Category 2—High Priority
Admission within one month is required for a condition that is causing significant pain, disability or has the potential to deteriorate quickly to the point that it may become urgent.

Category 3—Standard Priority
Admission should be provided within a reasonable time for a condition causing some pain, dysfunction or disability but which is not likely to deteriorate quickly or become an emergency. As far as possible, hospitals should aim to admit these patients within six months.[11]

You will have noticed that both pain and inherent condition feature in the assessment of need. Make a note for yourself about whether you agree with this classification of need. Also note that public hospitals can further divide these levels of priority, but must use this basic framework.

Category 4 of the Health Department's classification (not shown here), which allows for other social factors to influence the decision about the timing of admission, is closer to the distributive justice model. It takes into account the impact of social factors such as the ability to work, loss of income, level of support at home, and more.[12]

The modern application of distributive justice often takes comparative justice one step further. It allocates resources not just on need, but on what our society regards as an appropriate distribution of benefits and burdens. Distributive justice is really just the broad societal consensus on how to allocate rights, duties, and burdens among community members.[13] The important point is that burden is distributed according to the ability of sections of society to cope with it, and benefit is given to sections of society that need or deserve it. This means that need is not the only deciding factor. There is also some sort of social assessment of worth and deservedness going on here. If Rawls's model is applied in this assessment, then 'distribution' is interpreted as 'justice as fairness' or 'equality'. In distributive justice, any social difference can be the discriminating feature that decides whether or not a service will be provided, or at what level it will be supplied. For example, resources could go to the wealthy, if we judge they deserve it, and less to minority groups. Or the wealthy could be asked to bear more cost burden for the same care. The distinctions made between different social groups highlight the contemporary political and social divisions of the society that applies this justice model. You may like to read some of the ethical theories in Chapter 10 to help you decide how best to make a societal judgement on who deserves what treatment.

Applying the three models of justice

Once a system is in place, and is mandated by the institution in which you work, the real question for you, as a professional health care worker, is what discretion you have in applying that model. When professionals disagree violently with the model that seems to be operating, they may decide to protest. Our health care history is replete with examples of professionals protesting about the amount of resources provided to them to get their job done, or about the way in which some types of treatment seem to be undertaken (or some clients treated) but not others. Client groups too can voice dissatisfaction with how resources are shared, how some treatments are developed and others not, and about how long it seems to take for their health care needs to be met. A case study of the potential availability of new drugs has been included in the following section, 'The business of provision', for you to consider the issue of resource development in a practical treatment context.

THE BUSINESS OF PROVISION

Being in the business of providing health care involves charging money and buying human, and other, resources. In Australia, we have Medicare, a Commonwealth system that covers basic medical consultations, basic pathology services, and public provision of health care in public hospitals. Medicare pays health service providers with money collected from

Commonwealth income taxes. Providers are paid predetermined amounts for each service they provide. The services for which patients are covered under Medicare are tightly defined under the Medicare Benefits Schedule. What is included changes from time to time.

The following is an example of how a Medicare rebate can change. In the late 1990s, the following new condition was placed on the granting of a rebate offered in relation to a particular psychiatric condition: 'it is not sufficient for the patient's illness to fall within the diagnostic criteria. It must be evident that a significant level of impairment exists which interferes with the patient's quality of life'.[14] Changes to what services are covered, and to what extent, can also be driven by budget considerations. Also implemented at the same time was a restriction on the availability of benefits for the removal of broadly classified skin lesions. This change was due to a '30% increase in Medicare outlays above that anticipated'.[15] The rebates that are publicly funded are altered from time to time so that areas of need are balanced with areas of demand, to ensure equitable distribution of public funds.

Some health care practitioners choose to only charge the Medicare rebate, which is 75 to 85 per cent of the scheduled fee for any particular service (depending on the provider and where the service is received). These providers are termed 'bulk-billers': their service is largely paid for by Commonwealth Medicare funds.

Medicare is set up so that medical care is available when needed (and to a reasonable level) without financial considerations impeding that care. Providers can enter bulk-billing agreements with the government, ensuring that no money changes hands between the patient and provider. The number of providers prepared to bulk-bill has fallen dramatically over the last few years, to the point where the Federal government is considering a bonus scheme for GPs who bulk-bill patients in vulnerable groups.[16] Medicare is not meant to be used in instances when compensation may be claimed, and when medical bills will effectively be the responsibility of the person who caused the injury to the other person. One exception is provided for motor vehicle accidents (MVAs), where compensation or insurance claims may be routinely sought. The scheme for MVAs involves a separate bulk-billing arrangement so that ambulance officers arriving on the scene of an accident need not worry about who will pay for the service. The bill is worked out later, making it possible to institute essential care and transport to hospital immediately.[17] Emergency departments receive MVA casualties with the same expectations.

While Medicare is federally budgeted, state governments have their own budgets to run hospitals and to provide numerous other community and public health services. Both state and federal government budgets are routinely available, when tabled in Parliament, and they give an insight into what the current government's key objectives are in delivering health care, and how money is spent to achieve those objectives. Debating a budget for a service makes little sense unless the good that is trying to be achieved is also discussed.

The following exercise illustrates the breadth of one state government's health department budget. This exercise demonstrates the difficult budget decisions that must be made when resources become even more limited than usual, or when primary objectives change. Inevitably, some services lose money as that money is shifted to other services or is cut from the budget entirely. This is a macro exercise: it steps away from individual treatment decisions and asks you to think about what resources the system, or large service units, have at their disposal. Once budget cuts or rearrangements are instituted, those running the services have to: examine the objectives of the service; agree on how best to distribute what they have; and more fundamentally, decide whether they can still provide the 'good' that they believe they are there to provide.

Exercise 2.2 Budgets and priority decisions

This exercise uses the budget of the New South Wales Department of Health and the stated programs for achieving the objectives of the budget, as published in the parliamentary paper 'Budget Paper No 3' for 2002–03.[18] Examine the budget and consider the ministerial directive that priorities should change slightly. Think about how to achieve these changes in priority without allocating additional money. You may move money, but not add more. Before you start, put a 'hat' on, and adopt the role of stakeholder. Stakeholder roles can include health professionals (for example, doctors, nurses, and others), consumers of health services/clients (for example, patient advocates, particular client groups), planners (for example, chief executive officers, government representatives), and the general community (for example, local councils, mothers groups). You may be able to think of other stakeholders as well. This stakeholder exercise is fun in a tutorial or lecture format, with the groups not only implementing the ministerial directive, but also bringing their own agendas to the budget rearrangement.

The hypothetical ministerial directive for this exercise is that aged care and Aboriginal disease prevention programs should be a focus in the coming year, and that operations that can be achieved in day surgery should be carried out in that setting rather than with pre- and post-operation overnight stays.

A budget rearrangement can be combined with the additional scenario of a forthcoming pay increase for nurses, and a pay decrease for visiting medical officers (a similar exercise is found in Mitchell and Lovat's book *Bioethics for Medical and Health Professionals*).[19] This exercise asks you to find out the objectives of each program, and the good each is aiming for, and to consider them before budgets are rearranged. The detailed objectives can be found in the parliamentary papers referred to in Mitchell and Lovat's example, and the summary objectives are reproduced for you under each budget item.

Some health care workers are very uncomfortable about justice decisions being made as part of treatment decisions about individual clients, others less so. It could be argued that the duty to care for the individual client is paramount, and therefore should not be subject to broad budgetary discussions. On the other hand, with a limited resource, health professionals' obligations are also to other potential clients whom they have not yet met, but who might walk through the door and need treatment in the near future. That is why professional codes of ethics emphasise duty to society as well as duty to the individual client, as we saw in Chapter 1. The modern business of health care forces you to consider others as well as those whose health needs are right in front of you.

Budget exercise	
New South Wales Department of Health, Total Expenses Budget 2002–03	$000
Ambulatory, primary, and (general) community-based services **Primary and community-based services**	731 356
program objective: 'to improve, maintain or restore health through health promotion, early intervention, assessment, therapy and treatment services for clients in a home or community setting'.	
program description: 'provision of health services to persons attending community health centres or in the home, including health promotion activities, community based women's health, dental, drug and alcohol and HIV/AIDS services. Provision of grants to Non-Government Organisations for community health purposes'.[20]	
Aboriginal health services	29 658
program objective: 'to raise the health status of Aborigines and promote a healthy life style'.	
program description: 'provision of supplementary health services to Aborigines, particularly in the areas of health promotion, health education and disease prevention. (Note: This program excludes most services for Aborigines provided directly by area and district health services and other general health services which are used by all members of the community)'.[21]	
Outpatient services	808 160
program objective: 'to improve, maintain or restore health, through diagnosis, therapy, education and treatment services for ambulant patients in a hospital setting.'	
program description: 'provision of services provided in outpatient clinics including low level emergency care, diagnostic and pharmacy services and radiotherapy treatment'.[22]	
Acute health services **Emergency services**	791 591
program objective: 'to reduce the risk of premature death and disability for people suffering injury or acute illness by providing timely emergency diagnostic, treatment and transport services'.	
program description: 'provision of emergency road and air ambulance services and treatment of patients in designated emergency departments of public hospitals'.[23]	

Overnight acute inpatient services	3 446 381
program objective: 'to restore or improve health, and manage risks of illness, injury and childbirth through diagnosis and treatment for people intended to be admitted to hospital on an overnight basis'.	
program description: 'provision of health care to patients admitted to public hospitals with the intention that their stay will be overnight, including elective surgery and maternity services'.[24]	
Same-day acute inpatient services	485 940
program objective: 'to restore or improve health and manage risks of illness, injury and childbirth through diagnosis and treatment for people intended to be admitted to hospital and discharged on the same day'.	
program description: 'provision of health care to patients who are admitted to public hospitals with the intention that they will be admitted, treated and discharged on the same day'.[25]	
Mental health services	623 494
program objective: 'to improve the health, well being and social functioning of people with disabling mental disorders and to reduce the incidence of suicide, mental health problems and mental disorders in the community.'	
program description: 'provision of an integrated and comprehensive network of services by area health services and community based organisations for people affected by mental illness and mental health problems. The development of preventative programs which meet the needs of specific client groups'.[26]	
Rehabilitation and extended care services	897 404
program objective: 'to improve or maintain the well-being and independent functioning of people with disabilities or chronic conditions, the frail aged and the terminally ill'.	
program description: 'provision of appropriate health care services for persons with long term physical and psycho-physical disabilities and for the frail-aged. Coordination of the Department's services for the aged and disabled with those provided by other agencies and individuals'.[27]	
Population and community-based services	201 646
program objective: 'to promote health and reduce the incidence of preventable disease and disability by improving access to opportunities and prerequisites for good health'.	
program description: 'provision of health services targeted at broad population groups including environmental health protection, food and poisons regulation and monitoring of communicable diseases'.[28]	
Teaching and research	328 330
program objective: 'to develop the skills and knowledge of the health workforce to support patient care and population health. To extend knowledge through scientific enquiry and applied research aimed at improving the health and well-being of the people of New South Wales'.	
program description: 'provision of professional training for the needs of the New South Wales health system. Strategic investment in research and development to improve the health and well being of the people of New South Wales'.[29]	

In the United Kingdom, in the context of limited resources, rationing and managed care, and therefore limitations on the funds available to specific regions, have been a reality for over ten years. While there are many forms of managed care, in essence it involves reducing health care costs by directing funds for specific services, or for particular patient communities, towards certain health care providers who are able to provide those services at below a designated cost. The health carer is usually limited in what he or she can decide to offer the client, as the person managing the care (the person responsible for carrying out government policy) looks to all the services likely to be needed before imposing budgetary restrictions. The physician is not routinely the budget holder or managed-care coordinator (the person who keeps an eye on the budget and assesses the competing claims on the resources). Most general practitioners can only choose to be budget holders if their practice is of a sufficient size; for example, if they are large-scale purchasers of health services (such as acute services or specialist services), and are prominent as primary-care providers (relative to those acute and specialist services).[30] Of course, not all GPs want this funding responsibility. There is an ongoing concern that the United Kingdom system still harbours inequality.[31] The UK dentists are included in the public rebate NHS system, unlike Australia. Yet, they are increasingly electing not to accept new NHS patients on their practice lists. So, care is on a private basis, with the patient paying the full dental care bill to the dentist. The 'opening' of a list to public patients now prompts local media coverage.[32]

How a system is funded and structured can challenge the way individual health care workers relate to clients, as has been debated in New Zealand, where budget holding has been trialled. At the heart of the debate is the professional need to have good, coordinated information available, and to protect clients and client interests in an increasingly competitive environment.[33]

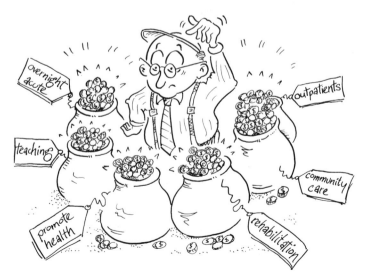

Different models of managed care in the USA can place the rationing decision with one primary provider, usually medical or nursing staff, who then coordinates his or her own service provision with the services of other professionals. A number of models that help determine who should exercise that rationing decision have been proposed. In all these models, the value of the personal provider–client relationship remains extremely important.[34] That relationship clearly faces new challenges, including threats posed to the trust that clients place in their carer, as the professional strives for the best possible care for all clients under their ambit and care.

Asch and Ubel have also described the way that, under the managed care system operating in the USA, doctors are forced to take responsibility for choosing the cheapest treatment that accords with the 'standard of care' set by the managed care policy. They describe how the government 'caps' (puts a limit on) the costs of particular services; this forces the physician to think beyond the individual client, appeal to the 'standard of care' (which, in most cases, is the most commonly used treatment rather than the best), and finally, make do with less than the best, unless other options have failed.[35] A vignette by Asch and Ubel was written to demonstrate how the most reliable option is often the last considered because it is the most expensive. This vignette could be used for discussion in class. Any routine normal treatment could be substituted to make the vignette appropriate for particular professions.

Ms Cooper sees her general internist, Dr Kelley, about her seasonal allergies. Dr Kelley explains that although he believes a nonsedating antihistamine is likely to be better tolerated, he thinks it is reasonable to try a less expensive conventional antihistamine first and to use the more expensive kind only if Ms Cooper is troubled by sedation.[36]

Note your list of the goods achieved for the client, and for the other potential clients in this scenario.

....

....

....

....

....

....

....

....

Exercise 2.3 Primary care decisions

Now try the following exercise:

GPs in a budget holding context in the UK are encouraged to prescribe generic drugs rather than brand names whenever possible. Those prescribing brand names consistently are 'visited' by representatives of the budget team for their area, to try and encourage more cost-effective patterns of prescribing.

What should the GPs be asked to do, and what should the GPs' response be? Try to set out your reasons, and explain them to a fellow colleague or friend.

In Thailand, there has been controversy over the 30-baht health care scheme, in which patients pay this small amount (approx $1.50 Australian, and 0.90¢ US) for each treatment, and then the local hospital covers all further treatment costs. When referral to tertiary care specialist or intensive treatment facilities for complex or chronic conditions is likely to be costly, there is reportedly reluctance by some local hospitals to refer.[37]

In Australia, the Commonwealth Government has trialed coordinated care to test the hypothesis that 'by breaking down these [service providers] barriers and maximising funding and service flexibility, in conjunction with an agreed and co-ordinated care plan, the health and well-being of these people can be improved for any given dollar input'.[38] The trials are focusing on care management and budget coordination for high-service clients, such as elderly persons with dementia, who are unable to manage their own care in the current system. The focus was on complex and chronic conditions, which, by their nature, consume enormous amounts of the health budget. The coordination of different services provided promising results in the first trials, and a second round of trials is underway for people with chronic asthma, diabetes and heart conditions, as well as for people in Aboriginal communities with chronic disease issues. The trials are expected to run to 2004.[39]

In the UK, US, and Australian systems, with their different approaches to budgeted health care, the notion of managing resources rather than just providing care will take some time for the health carers to come to terms with.[40]

In the USA, a managed care system is quite common, as many patients are insured with managed care providers. Hospitals can be nominated as care providers by insurers, and they negotiate contracts for reimbursement for care provided. These contract negotiations can be heated and difficult, as hospitals seek to ensure they have sufficient funds to properly cover anticipated care costs. The large US government-funded plan for very low income earners (Medicare) used to provide a buffer for hospitals as contracted care providers. Now there is a context of falling Medicare rates, tighter margins with insurance contracts, and continuing backlash against managed care.[41] Practices can be nominated as providers of 'capitation contracts' to provide care for certain insured people. The physician needs to balance care and care costs—both those generated in a setting and those outsourced through referral. When asked about their practice in a managed care setting for a study in the USA, many expressed concerns about:

- the request for referral or use of outside care
- when to authorise treatments that would help, perhaps more 'socially' than medically
- patients' requests for specific treatments which may be expensive and which may require specific criteria to justify the expense under a managed care plan
- feeling a pressure to provide services outside own level of expertise, and
- wanting to give additional service, advice, or supply of goods for free, but feeling obliged to limit expenses for the sake of the practice.[42]

Many of these concerns are about trying to contain costs and services in one setting. This is a common theme in different country's settings. The limited referral process, or more strictly controlled and budgeted referral process, means waiting lists and longer waiting times for patients to access those secondary services.

Working in managed care brings decisions like drug prescriptions, hospital admission, referrals, and affiliated resource use into sharp focus. The 'budgets' that have to be balanced can be at area level, or in the US system, at insure coverage level. The different style of practice implicit in this organisation of care delivery is now taught in resident training in the USA. The case discussions during rounds involve clinical issues, but also issues of referral which could lead to resource use problems. Use of expensive procedures and specialty referrals are scrutinised.[43] This is clearly a different style of practice to that focused solely on maximal care of individuals using any or all available technology and resources.

The care received in hospitals is constantly assessed. Legislation in mid 2003 set required patient–nurse ratios for Californian hospitals. While care units can vary between three to ten patients per nurse, the aim is for an average of six patients per nurse. This follows research which shows that a higher nurse ratio and subsequently better surveillance of a patient's condition, leads to lower mortality figures and better job satisfaction for the nurses.[44] Human resources are as much in the debate about expenditure as procedural or treatment resources, as your budget exercise showed.

In the UK, waiting list systems for treatment in budgeted categories of care are causing exasperation at local levels. Children, for instance, may have changed significantly by the time their appointment for assessment of particular problems arrives. A qualitative interview study of access to cardiac rehabilitation services in an area of socio-economic deprivation in the UK demonstrated that waiting times were lengthy, and many people slipped through the care net due to limited service capacity and difficulties in accessing hospital based services from small towns. The patients and their families experienced frustration at still being on rehabilitation waiting lists sometimes months after cardiac episodes. Some people avoided the public system queue for services in the NHS by seeking out specific advice or using private rehabilitation services.[45] The government is tackling the waiting list delays in a number of ways. For hospitals, the ratings received for care and waiting times partly determine funding for those hospitals. Patients have a significant input into the ratings, with large scale patient surveys of care received in acute care and outpatient settings, being conducted regularly and the results incorporated into the ratings. In one survey program, 59 000 patients in NHS acute trusts and 123 000 patients in primary care trusts were involved in rating services.[46] This rating system is itself debated, but seems to be here to stay.

The managed care system, however it is formulated in each country, relies on 'trust' that pursuing the best possible care for each patient is the shared aim of the carer, the health service, and the funder. Managed care members interviewed by researchers have spoken about how important it is to have trust in the doctor, and also trust in the hospital, and now, trust in the insurer that best possible care will be made available.[47]

There are tools that can be used to decide if a service is worth offering, and if the society can afford to make it available. These tools focus on the likely benefit of the service, and then compare the benefit with the likely demand for the service, and the drain on available resources that offering the resource or service would cause.

Two of these tools are cost-effectiveness analysis, and cost–benefit analysis. Cost–benefit analysis compares the cost of a program with the expected benefits in dollars. The way that this analysis quantifies outcomes as hard currency makes it controversial in health. It is hard to quantify how much an improvement in health or lifestyle, or life years, means in real dollars. Cost-effectiveness analysis compares alternative ways of achieving a specific set of objectives or outcomes. Cost-effectiveness analysis is being increasingly used to decide program rationing in large health systems, such as in the US system. Its ethics are also being examined.

Exercise 2.4 Preventive testing budgets

A paper by Ubel, DeKay, Baron, and Asch reported on a study that posed the following scenario to experts in medical ethics and medical decision making.[48] Consider their scenario. What do you think should happen?

The federal government has set up a program to test for colon cancer in people enrolled in Medicaid, a government program that offers health insurance to low-income people and their families. The test allows doctors to find colon cancer at an early stage. So far, the federal government has offered the test to people at high risk for colon cancer, and this has prevented many of them from dying of colon cancer. Now the government wants to offer the test to the rest of the people receiving Medicaid, all of whom are at equally low risk for colon cancer.

A group of doctors was formed to help the government decide which of two tests to offer the low-risk people. Test 1 is inexpensive but does not always detect cancers in their early stages. Test 2 is more expensive but is better at detecting early cancers. The decision is complicated by budget limitations: the government has only a certain amount of money available to pay for the screening tests. After evaluating the costs and benefits of each test, the doctors have reached the following conclusions. The budget is just large enough to offer test 1 to all the low-risk people. With this approach, everyone can receive the test, and 1000 deaths from colon cancer will be prevented. The budget is just large enough to offer test 2 to half the low-risk people. With this approach, half the people can receive the test and half cannot, and 1100 deaths from colon cancer will be prevented.

The ethicists and decision makers who thought about this problem were told that the persons selected for screening, if the second scenario were to be followed (test 2 is offered to half the low-risk people), would be randomly selected on the basis of their social-security numbers. The ethicists who responded to the survey were uneasy about the assumption underpinning cost-effectiveness analysis: that 'it is best to maximize the total benefit per dollar spent, even if this is achieved by offering a health care intervention to only a portion of a population that might benefit from it'. They rejected the more effective test, in favour of making a test equally available to all potential recipients.[49] In doing so they implicitly challenged the utilitarian basis of cost-effectiveness analysis (achieving the greatest good for the greatest number).

....

....

....

....

....

....

....

....

One critic of this hypothetical has pointed out that it does not consider the possibility of moving money across from other budgets to be able to deliver a better test to all the low-income Medicaid recipients.[50]

This alternative is really the process, which was outlined for you earlier in this section, of rearranging budgets and budget priorities on a large scale.

The controversy associated with tools such as cost–benefit analysis and cost-effectiveness analysis is the way it requires decision makers to make value judgements about who, or what groups of people, should receive treatments. Its controversial nature also stems from the fact that the decision of worth is made before the actual consumer or patient enters the treatment context. The decision is made at a different time (for example, when setting up the service) or is made hypothetically (for example, for the type of situation that any given patient might, one day, be in).

An early experiment in limiting the costs of public programs was conducted in Oregon in the USA. Before decisions were made about how many of certain types of services should be offered to public patients, the community was asked to rate how successful these services were in adding quality life-years. The Oregon experiment in consultative rationing has been discussed at length elsewhere. The controversial aspects—such as making health-outcome or quality life-years the focus, considering the worth of the expected life-span, and making assumptions about the worth of health care programs—have also been debated. Kitzhaber and Kemmy, who were key figures in the Oregon experiment, describe their personal experience of the budget dilemma they were faced with:

> In the interim spring of 1986, a variety of factors combined to produce a budget shortfall of $35 million, and the E-Board took steps to bring the budget back into balance—among them, a decision to drop over 4300 Oregonians from state medical coverage
>
> … Not many months later, however, some of those human consequences began showing up in my emergency room—people who had delayed seeking timely treatment because they now had no way to pay for it.[51]

There is now a readiness to learn from the Oregon decisions. Despite the controversy surrounding it, it was one of the first social programs to acknowledge the limitations that health budgets pose to the goal of achieving health for all.

The above discussion focuses on the decisions involved in making a service available. The development of the service is also crucial.

PHARMACEUTICALS AND THE DEVELOPMENT OF NEW DRUGS

When you treat people, you look at what you can do, and you look at what is available as a resource to use in that management process or treatment process. Because new approaches and new treatments are constantly being developed, you need to keep up to date with professional literature to be able to make an informed assessment. This section looks at the development of new drugs. It is about the potential availability of a particular 'good'.

The development of new drugs is of tremendous ethical and social importance. It is fired by a need to find better ways of helping people with health problems, from niggling problems to minor episodic illnesses and chronic illnesses, and right through to serious and life-threatening conditions. The development of new drugs involves a massive human-resources commitment and substantial financial investment. It relies on government policy to provide both incentives and restraints (the latter for ethical purposes). More and more, the development of new drugs is being scrutinised and lobbied by patient advocates, and is increasingly attracting the scrutiny of social scientists and ethicists.

Given the political, economic, and social forces involved in drug development, it is not surprising that the objectives and guidelines of policy surrounding this issue change from time to time. Australia provides us with a clear example of this, particularly in relation to regulations for the evaluation of new drugs. The regulations seek to provide a balance between benefit and risk, with the latter including the health risks posed to participants in any trial of the drug prior to its release. The resources available to support the development of the drug, and its eventual availability, are considered, as is the worth of the project. In its consideration of all these factors, drug evaluation illustrates many of the key features of resources and justice debates.

The information that the health department has typically sought in its evaluations has been extremely wide ranging, including pharmaceutical, chemical, animal, pharmacological, and toxicological data (as well as clinical experience). In other words, they tend to ask for basic scientific information and information on the drug's application in the clinical context. The department relies heavily on skilled scientists to assess the information. This system has developed gradually, taking shape from 1970 when Commonwealth legislation was revised to give the minister for health the power to issue permits for the importation of drugs (based on an analysis of the drug's quality, efficacy, and safety). Before that, the focus of the legislation was predominantly on the quality of manufacture of the drug, and on ruling out the likelihood that it posed severe and life-threatening risks.[52]

A number of factors were influential in the change of thinking about new drugs that occurred in the 1960s. You may know some of these influencing factors. One particular Australian incident has been extremely important, in the overall context of Western health care, in bringing home to us the potential danger of seemingly routine drugs. Thalidomide, an apparently harmless and effective morning-sickness drug, was eventually found to be linked to physical deformities in the children of mothers who took the drug. This discovery resulted in tighter drug-evaluation systems in Australia and all around the world.

The focuses of Australian drug evaluation are now not only efficacy, safety, and quality, but also timely availability. In the quest for timely availability of new drugs, the drug-evaluation system has started to change rapidly. Just as thalidomide made a difference in the 1960s, there is now consensus that AIDS (acquired immunodeficiency syndrome), and the dearth of adequate treatments for the condition, has made a substantial difference to the current drug-regulation and evaluation system. Groups lobbying on behalf of AIDS patients have been campaigning for a drug regulation system that 'maximises the safety and efficacy of treatments, while at the same time expedites access to those treatments'.[53] Summary data to support the drug being registered is permitted, and human research ethics committees are relied on for assessment of research proposals for drug trials in humans. Ethics committees must ask: does the proposed benefit justify the risk, and if so, how much risk? Further, they need to consider whether it is acceptable to expose human participants to this risk, and other potential risks, before it is known whether the treatment will in fact work.

The decision process in HRECs, or human research ethics committees, formerly known as IECs, or institutional ethics committees, is the subject of further discussion in Chapter 9. The main job of these committees is to consider the ethics of research. They do so under the mandate of, but independently from, the institution in which the research is to be conducted, and they are guided by the NHMRC *National Statement on Ethical Conduct in Research Involving Humans*.[54] The committees rarely have basic scientists—such as chemists, physicists, biologists, or pharmacologists—on board, and some committee members feel uncertain about their relatively new role in considering drugs and drug trials with human participants. The ethical challenge now may be to provide these committees with the support and expert advice they need to make a reasonable risk–benefit assessment of drugs, and to continue to protect the safety and welfare of human participants in research.

Drug production is a business, conducted by companies who need to turn a profit to sustain the business and investment. There is tremendous pressure for drugs to be provided cheaply once they are proven effective. Whether the pharmaceutical industry can be a medicine provider, particularly in less developed countries, is a matter of debate. The business invests large amounts of money years in advance of any anticipated return on new drugs. Many generic drugs are produced cheaply once patents expire, and governments support subsidy of essential drugs in their own countries. The issue has been heatedly debated in the African context of high HIV rates and impoverishment of large affected communities.[55]

WHO has expressed its own optimal guidelines for the development of drugs and their testing in the approval process.[56] They recognise that some countries have more stringent guidelines than others, and propose minimum requirements for size and duration of trials, designed to ensure that adverse events will be picked up in both the trial and the monitoring system, which continues to safeguard people even when a drug is approved. These guidelines are meant to apply across national boundaries so that trials are of a high safety standard, even when countries do not have their own requirements. It is aimed at a basic protection, regardless of country, as is consistent with WHO's universal view of health promotion, which was reviewed earlier in this chapter. However, with the fifth revision of the Declaration of Helsinki in 2000, a balance between setting ethical standards and not prohibiting research in developing countries was revisited. New treatments now need not be tested against placebos, but preferably compared with the best available treatment, so that control group participants received some treatment where possible. The 'available treatments' are considered relevant to each context. Put simply, different treatments are readily available in different countries, and drug companies may not be required to ensure the same treatment standard for a comparison group in different countries.[57] This could theoretically lead to lesser standards if the available treatment is being applied to developing world research.

Whether such a double standard is ethically acceptable is heatedly debated. Kottow suggests that the eventual criticism of the infamous Willowbrook vaccine test research on institutionalised children and the Tuskegee syphilis progression research on largely black American impoverished men were two examples of local conditions finally not being judged as ethically acceptable. He argues strongly not to allow different standards to be used in international drug trials.[58] A further revision of the Declaration, was still under discussion in late 2003 by the World Medical Association. This would potentially qualify responsibilities of doctors to deliver best proven treatments when they were not available in particular contexts, both within trial protocols and after the trials had been completed.[59]

The debate on the acceptable balance between risk and potential benefit in developing new drugs continues in Australia, and is likely to continue worldwide as well. This debate is at the heart of research (research is discussed further in Chapter 9). The key question is what risk is reasonable in the quest for new or better ways of providing health care.

This debate is, in some ways, also a debate about autonomy and beneficence. It is recognised that where no proven treatments are available, there is a place for the exercise of patient choice, and drugs and drug trials can be fast-tracked to allow that choice. However, there is an underlying limit to the amount of risk that people can choose to expose themselves to, and that limit is the willingness of professionals to help them. It is increasingly recognised that there is a limit to the amount of resources that can be committed to trying unproven treatments. Each proposal for increased patient participation and choice in drug trials is debated on the grounds of appropriate choice, and appropriate risk.

The trend towards patient choice may have been carried to extremes, especially in the case of a serious, infectious, and life-threatening condition such as HIV and the resulting AIDS-defining conditions (illnesses indicating that a patient's HIV has progressed to AIDS). Towards the mid

1990s, the pendulum of professional opinion slowly swung back towards limited client choice to undertake risk, and a greater emphasis began to be placed on safety and reliable results.

Drug regulation illustrates how fluid the debate over acceptable risk and objective benefit is. The debate can swing depending on context, perceived threat, and available resources. It is also constructed differently by different groups. To groups lobbying on behalf of those with AIDS, more risk in trying unproven treatments may be acceptable. To health professionals, a conservative risk would be preferable. If our society had virtually limitless funds, or if our society trusted entirely that individuals could choose their own best path in medical treatment, there is no doubt that the balance between, on the one hand, personal choice, and on the other, safety and reliability would be quite different.[60]

PATIENTS/CLIENTS AS CONSUMERS

The person who uses, or is likely to use, a health service is a consumer. More and more, consumers are regarded as active participants in health care. This is so in two senses: in the sense of being actively involved, as clients, in individual treatment decisions; and in the sense of having an impact on the design and operation of a health service. Their views on health care are valued. Their views are valuable in alerting health care workers to the primary concerns and feelings of clients as they (the clients) negotiate the health care system.

A study of consumer perspectives on illness has been carried out in the Netherlands by de Ridder, Depla, Severens, and Malsch. These researchers used 'concept mapping' and discussion with consumers who had chronic disease. They found that consumers used two different dimensions to describe how they coped with illness: coping with the illness, and coping with the health care system. In coping with the illness, autonomy and acceptance of the illness featured strongly. In coping with the health care system, a 'professional relationship with the physician based on mutual trust and respect between two equal partners' was emphasised.[61]

You will find these themes—client autonomy, acceptance of illness on the part of clients, and health worker–client relationships based on trust and respect—throughout this book. When a person falls ill, or has a need for a health service, he or she is coming to terms with that illness or need, and is, at the same time, entering a health service and seeking your help. This same study also makes a distinction between the modern consumer, who makes demands and is assertive, and the traditional model of the client, who feels powerless and relies heavily on trust.[62] There are different types of consumers. Some researchers question whether clients want to be involved in decision making. This is a separate issue from whether clients want to be informed.[63]

Whether people are 'entitled' to have the goods that their society offers is often hotly debated. This is, in essence, a debate over whether people are entitled to consume the goods or services available. It is squarely a justice issue. Sometimes services are not so much pursued by consumers, as promoted by society. For instance, there is currently a government health program with the objective of increasing the number of children in Australia who are immunised against basic diseases such as whooping cough, measles, and rubella. The rationale for this program was that immunisation rates have been falling, and the incidence of death or serious illness among children who contract these diseases is rising.

A precis of the immunisation debate has been written by Michael Walsh. The focus of this paper is whether or not individuals should be able to decide to accept this service. Walsh argues that individuals should have a right to assess the benefits and risks of the immunisation program for themselves. The relatively small number of serious side-effects from vaccines may be more significant for some people than others, and poses a difficult dilemma for parents, as they try to balance their parental and societal responsibilities.[64] Can individuals make this choice themselves, or has the choice been made at a societal level? Are the patients (or their parents) active consumers, or, by virtue of living in society, has immunising your child become a non-negotiable responsibility?

Dr John Yu, a prominent former administrator of the new Children's Hospital at Westmead, has suggested that people who place others at risk by refusing such services should be denied other (non-health related) state benefits. The following article in the *Sydney Morning Herald* had this to say about Yu's views:

> Yu says, crusader-like, that the failure to immunise is a violation of a child's rights. 'No parents have a right to deny a child's safety,' he says. He maintains we have the lowest rate of immunisation of any country in the Asia-Pacific region. In many of these countries, immunisation is imposed and he would like some draconian steps to be taken here. 'It's very simple. Nobody should receive child endowment or other benefits unless their child is fully immunised. If you accept the benefits of the State, you must accept your obligation to the community at large.'[65]

As a revision of this chapter, try this exercise with a group of fellow health workers, or with a group of students. Pick a good that your profession offers, and trace its development and availability. This will make you examine what your profession sees as a good, and how the potential for achieving that good is balanced against, on the one hand, possible harms, and on the other, the need to gather and deploy the resources necessary to aid its development and accessibility. As you find out about your good, think about what it means for your commitment, as a health care professional, to the principles of caring, doing no harm, respecting autonomy, and fair distribution. You may find that the relative emphasis you place on each of these will change.

We have grown used to looking back on earlier health care as particularly paternalistic beneficence. We may look back on the 1980s as the decade of autonomy. In the 1990s our enthusiasm for patient and client autonomy has been tempered. The kind of beneficence practised by health care professionals is increasingly limiting available client choices, as the health care professions and the surrounding regulatory system impose limits on client wishes, according to which wishes they are comfortable with and are able to grant. In the modern health care context of stretched resources, and fluctuating financial situations, justice concerns may well be the issue that will dominate health care ethics in this century.[66]

Summary of key issues

- Institutional goals and values
- Defining a good to aim for
- Development of goods
- Sharing limited resources
- Interests and rights
- Justice models: justice as fairness, comparative justice, distributive justice
- Balancing risks and benefits for clients and others

Notes

1 For example, in summaries such as Australian Bureau of Statistics, *Private Hospitals 1994–95*, no. 4390.0; Australian Bureau of Statistics, *Hospitals Australia 1991–92*, no. 4391.10; and Smith & Nephew Surgical, *Hospital and Health: Services Year Book 1995/96*, 20th edn, Peter Isaacson Publications Pty Ltd, 1995/96.

2 J. S. Mill, 'On Liberty', in *Three Essays*, Oxford University Press, London, 1975, pp. 92–114.

3 M. J. Bossuyt, *Guide to the 'Travaux Preparatoires' of the International Covenant on Civil and Political Rights*, Martinus Nijhoff Publishers, Dordrecht, 1987.

4 J. W. Peabody, S. R. Bickel, and J. S. Lawson, 'The Australian Health Care System: Are the Incentives Down Under or Right Side Up?', *Journal of the Australian Medical Association*, vol. 276, no. 24, 1996, pp. 1944–50.

5 R. Gillon, *Philosophical Medical Ethics*, John Wiley & Sons, Chichester, 1986, pp. 54–8.

6 J. Devereux, *Medical Law: Text, Cases and Materials*, Cavendish, Sydney, 1997, p. 396.

7 D. Callahan, 'Achievable Goals', *World Health*, no. 5, 49th year, 1996, pp. 6–8.

8 Preamble to the constitution of WHO, in *WHO Basic Documents*, 26th edn, World Health Organization, Geneva, 1976, p. 1; and Dr J. W. Lee, Director-General Elect, Speech to the Fifty-sixth World Health Assembly, 21 May 2003, Geneva, Switzerland, at http://www.who.int/dg_elect/wha56_jwlspeech/en/print.html.

9 GDP figures presented here are from GDP figures compiled from a number of different sources, by Peabody, Bickel and Lawson, pp. 1944–50.

10 T. L. Beauchamp and J. F. Childress, *Principles of Biomedical Ethics*, 4th edn, Oxford University Press, New York, 1994, p. 340.

11 New South Wales Department of Health (Audit Branch), Hospital Booking List Clinical Priority Classification System (93/57), in *Patient Matters: Manual for Area Health Services and Public Hospitals*, New South Wales Department of Health, Sydney, June 1989 (updated regularly, and current as at 2003), section 12.11, 12.34, pp. 323–6.

12 New South Wales Department of Health (Audit Branch).

13 B. M. Dickens, 'Legal Approaches to Health Care Ethics and the Four Principles', in R. Gillon (ed.), *Principles of Health Care Ethics*, John Wiley & Sons, Chichester, United Kingdom,1994, p. 315.

14 Commonwealth Department of Health and Family Services, *Supplement to Medicare Benefits Schedule Book* of 1 November 1996, effective 1 May 1997, AGPS, p. 7.

15 Commonwealth Department of Health and Family Services, p. 3.

16 As detailed in the Budget for 2003–04, and outlined in the media release of April 2003. Senator the Hon. Kay Patterson, Minister for Health and Ageing. Media Release. *A fairer Medicare—better access, more affordable*. April 28, 2003.

17 Motor Accidents Authority, *New South Wales Health Bulk Billing Handbook*, State Health Publications no. (FB) 960105, Motor Accidents Authority Reorder No. RE 010796, May 1996.

18 Parliament of New South Wales, 'Budget Paper No. 3 Vol. 2', Budget Estimates 2002–03, Parliamentary Paper No. 97b of 2002, ordered to be printed 4 June 2002.

19 K. R. Mitchell and T. J. Lovat, *Bioethics for Medical and Health Professionals*, Social Sciences Press, Wentworth Falls, 1991, p. 136.

20 Parliament of New South Wales, pp. 8–20.

21 Parliament of New South Wales, pp. 8–21.

22 Parliament of New South Wales, pp. 8–22.

23 Parliament of New South Wales, pp. 8–23.

24 Parliament of New South Wales, pp. 8–25.

25 Parliament of New South Wales, pp. 8–27.

26 Parliament of New South Wales, pp. 8–28.

27 Parliament of New South Wales, pp. 8–30.

28 Parliament of New South Wales, pp. 8–32.

29 Parliament of New South Wales, pp. 8–35.

30 L. F. P. Smith and J. R. Morrissy, 'Ethical Dilemmas for General Practitioners under the UK New Contract', *Journal of Medical Ethics*, vol. 20, 1994, pp. 175–80; J. Pratt, 'Redefining the Core Values and Role of General Practice in the UK', *Education for Health*, vol. 10, no. 1, 1997, pp. 35–45.

31 'Health Inequality: The UK's Biggest Issue', editorial, *Lancet*, vol. 349, 1997, p. 1185.

32 P. Morris, 'County dental care is in crisis', *Gloucestershire Echo*, Friday July 18, 2003, pp. 1–2; P. Morris, 'Queueing for NHS dentists – is it Prestbury next?', *Gloucestershire Echo*, Wednesday July 30, 2003, p. 3.

33 New Zealand Medical Association Newsletter, no. 108, 1994, p. 3.

34 C. Urbina, A. Kaufman, and D. Derksen, 'The Managed Health Care Scenario: Challenges to Future Medical Training', *Education for Health*, vol. 10, no. 1, 1997, pp. 25–33.

35 D. A. Asch and P. A. Ubel, 'Rationing by Any Other Name', *New England Journal of Medicine*, vol. 336, no. 23, 1997, pp. 1668–71.

36 Asch and Ubel, p. 1670.

37 K. Lyall, '30-baht health care a fatal prescription', *The Australian*, Wednesday April 24, 2002, p. 8.

38 Commonwealth Department of Human Services and Health, Calls for Expressions of Interest in Conducting Trials in Coordinated Care, Commonwealth Department of Human Services and Health, Canberra, September 1995, p. 6.

39 Acute and Co-ordinated Care Branch, Commonwealth Department of Health and Ageing. Primary Care Initiatives: Further Co-ordinated Care Trials. 20 Nov 2000, at http://www.health.gov.au/hsdd/primcare/acoorcar/abtrials.htm.

40 A. G. Magney and C. A. Berglund, 'Co-ordinated care: ethics debate as part of the trial process', *Evaluation*, vol. 6, no. 4, 2000, pp. 455–69.

41 L. B. Benko, and D. Bellandi, 'The rough and tumble of it', *Modern Healthcare*, vol. 31, no. 12, 2001, pp. 53–4.

42 S. D. Pearson, J. E. Sabin, and T. Hyams, 'Caring for patients within a budget: physicians' tales from the front lines of managed care', *Journal of Clinical Ethics*, vol. 13, no. 2, 2002, pp. 115–23.

43 A. G. Gomez, C. T. Grimm, E. F. T. Yee, and S. A. Skootsky, 'Preparing residents for managed care practice using an experience-based curriculum', *Academic Medicine*, vol. 72, no. 11, 1997, pp. 959–65.

44 L. H. Aiken, S. P. Clarke, D. M. Sloane, J. Sochalski, and J. H. Silber, 'Hospital nurse staffing and patient mortality, nurse burnout, and job dissatisfaction', *Journal of the American Medical Association*, vol. 288, no. 16, 2002, pp. 1987–93.

45 A. M. Todd, E. A. Lacey, and F. McNeill, ''I'm still waiting…': barriers to accessing cardiac rehabilitation services', *Journal of Advanced Nursing*, vol. 40, no. 4, 2002, pp. 413–20.

46 Commission for Health Improvement, *National Patients Survey Programme: 2003 Results*, NHS, London, 2003, at http://www.chi.nhs.uk/eng/surveys/nps2003.

47 S. Dorr-Goold and G. Klipp, 'Managed care members talk about trust', *Social Science & Medicine*, vol. 54, no. 6, 2002, pp. 879–88.

48 P. A. Ubel, M. L. DeKay, J. Baron, and D. A. Asch, 'Cost-effectiveness Analysis in a Setting of Budget Constraints', *New England Journal of Medicine*, vol. 334, no. 18, 1996, pp. 1174–7.

49 Ubel et al., p. 1176.

50 J. S. McCombs, letter, *New England Journal of Medicine*, vol. 335, no. 19, 1996, p. 1465.

51 J. Kitzhaber and A. M. Kemmy, 'On the Oregon Trail', *British Medical Bulletin*, vol. 51, no. 4, 1995, p. 809.

52 *Therapeutic Goods Act 1966–73 (Cwlth)*, particularly section 29(1), *Therapeutic Goods Amendment Act 1991 (Cwlth)*, section 4.

53 Australian Federation of AIDS Organisations (AFAO), Submission to the Baume Review of the Drug Evaluation and Access Process in Australia, AFAO, May 1991, p. 4.

54 National Health and Medical Research Council, *National Statement on Ethical Conduct in Research Involving Humans*, Canberra, AGPS, 1999.

55 D. Henry and J. Lexchin, 'The pharmaceutical industry as a medicines provider', *The Lancet*, vol. 360, no. 9345, 2002, pp. 1590–2.

56 WHO, 'Documentation Requirements for Approval: Safety', *WHO Drug Information*, vol. 10, no. 4, 1996, pp. 180–1; and WHO, 'Drug Safety Monitoring Centres', *WHO Drug Information*, vol. 10, no. 4, 1996, p. 181.

57 World Medical Association, World Medical Association Declaration of Helsinki: *Ethical principles for medical research involving human subjects*. Ferney-Voltaire, World Medical Association, 2000; S. M. Tollman, 'Fair partnerships support ethical research', *British Medical Journal*, vol. 323, no. 7326, pp. 1417–25, at p. 1428.

58 M. H. Kottow, 'Who is my brother's keeper?', *Journal of Medical Ethics*, vol. 28, 2002, pp. 24–7, at p. 26.

59 World Medical Association, 'WMA to continue discussion on Declaration of Helsinki', Press release, 14 September 2003, at http://www.wma.net.

60 C. A. Berglund, 'Bioethics: A Balancing of Concerns in Context', *Australian Health Review*, vol. 20, no. 1, 1997, pp. 43–52.

61 D. de Ridder, M. Depla, P. Severens, and M. Malsch, 'Beliefs on Coping with Illness: A Consumer's Perspective', *Social Science & Medicine*, vol. 44, no. 5, 1997, pp. 553–9.

62 de Ridder et al., p. 557.

63 R. B. Deber, N. Kraetschmer, and J. Irvine, 'What Role do Patients Wish to Play in Treatment Decision Making?', *Archives of Internal Medicine*, vol. 156, 1996, pp. 1414–20.

64 M. Walsh, *The National Childhood Immunisation Campaign: Ethical Issues*, Issues Paper No. 3, Autumn 1997, The Australian Institute of Health Law & Ethics, Canberra, 1997.

65 A. Joel, 'The Man Who Cares for Kids', *Sydney Morning Herald: Good Weekend*, 4 January 1997, p. 25.

66 Berglund, pp. 43–52.

3

Enter the patient

Overview

- Meeting the patient/client
- The beginnings of treatment responsibility
- A dynamic relationship
- Negotiating treatment
- Seeking consent

This chapter focuses on the ethics involved in the immediate client–carer relationship, from the time the client enters the treatment context and becomes the carer's patient. In this chapter, the reader will grapple with the dynamic nature of the client–carer relationship. The individual client's input into their treatment is explored, and different approaches to negotiating treatment are discussed. Models ranging from paternalism to liberalism are examined, as are philosophical choices involved in information disclosure. Informed consent is a key focus.

MEETING THE PATIENT/CLIENT

When you meet a client for the first time, you meet a new person. A first rule of thumb is to try to respect people for who they are, not what you would like them to be.

We should try to respect everyone we meet, no matter who they are. If you were to make a list of how you could respect a person (and you could do this either alone or in a group), your list would probably include ideas on how you can respect or uphold that person's dignity, wishes, and integrity.

Exercise 3.1 People you meet

Take a moment to think about the last client, or person, whom you met. What did you notice about him or her? What did they tell you about themselves? What makes this person different from other people? What makes them them? What I noticed about the last client (person) I met was:

....

....

....

....

....

....

....

....

....

The principle of 'respect for persons', otherwise known as the principle of autonomy, is about respecting the wishes and dignity of each person. When asked to respond to the question 'How do you respect people?', many people would write down issues such as 'acknowledge them as people', 'listen to them', 'treat them with dignity', 'ask for and listen to their opinion', and 'give them privacy'. In practice, the principle of 'respect for persons' often revolves around individuals' freedom to plan and choose what will happen to them; that is, their right to be autonomous. Autonomy, derived from the Greek terms 'autos' and 'nomos', means self-rule. In the context of health care this refers, of course, to the client having a degree of power over treatment decisions. A frequent misunderstanding among students is that it is about professionals deciding what should be done in any given treatment situation. While there is such a thing as professional autonomy, generally, when the terms 'autonomy' or 'respect for persons' are used, they refer to client autonomy.

To be able to uphold people's autonomy, to uphold respect for persons, you need to know a little about them. But first, you need to put them at ease. Clients entering your health care service are likely to feel sick, or anxious, or scared, or all three. As a good professional, you should strive to put people at ease. Once you have done this you can begin to hear the client's story and understand them as a person. You need to know what has happened, what their symptoms feel like, what the client values, and what they would prefer. First things first: What is the problem? What brings them to a health care context?

The initial decision to tell others about private information, to allow someone to touch us to see what is wrong, and to tell others something that is personal is at the heart of health care. We all have different thresholds of privacy, as the following exercise demonstrates.

Exercise 3.2 Preferences for privacy

In a group, turn to the person next to you, and tell them a secret about yourself. Tell them something that you don't necessarily want everyone to know. Before you tell them, alert them to the sensitivity of the information by asking them not to tell anyone else. If you think of something but decide you really don't want to tell anyone, let them know you'd rather not say anything. Then, count how many people had a secret that they decided to tell, and that they therefore entrusted to their neighbour.

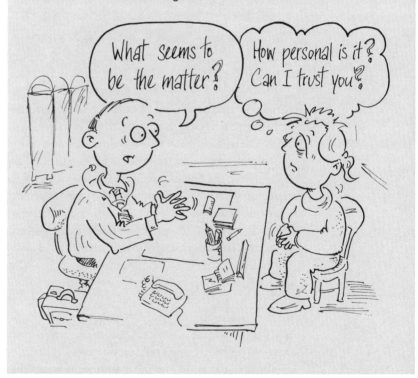

In your health care relationships, your patients make decisions all the time about what secrets to tell, what to let you see, and how much to trust you, the health care worker, to use that information constructively and to respect it as private and confidential.

The relationship between counsellor and client could be a useful way for you to think about meeting and getting to know your own clients or patients. A good counsellor–client relationship involves establishing trust and ground rules, before tackling the difficult issues that have prompted the client to seek counselling. The initial stages of a counselling relationship have been identified as follows: meeting the client, during which time both the counsellor and client are on their 'best behaviour'; discussion of surface issues, in which the client feels able to discuss everyday issues; and then revelation of deeper issues, which occurs in the context of a developed relationship in which the client feels confident and trusts the counsellor. The counsellor's skill is in setting the client at ease through the initial stage, and gradually encouraging self-revelation.[1] It is a subtle art, and one that counsellors must master, as it is required for an ethical relationship with clients to develop. So much depends on understanding both your client and the problem at hand. You may, like counsellors, have the luxury of more than one meeting to achieve this. If you don't, your bedside manner is all the more important.

A similar appreciation of privacy is expected in relation to physical body exposure. A practitioner becomes used to draping patients so as to expose only as much of their bodies as is necessary, and to letting patients dress and undress in as much privacy as is possible.

As clients disclose information and give you access to their personal thoughts and feelings, you are beginning to get to know them, and are trying to understand what has happened to them, and how serious it is. You tend to make running notes in your head about what you could do to help. You start a medical record, or add to one that has already been started. The initial records that you make about someone are a crucial piece in any treatment relationship. They should be accurate and complete; they can be initiated by or added to by any health care worker; and they become the basis of noting and assessing progress as the client is engaged in treatment.

Health departments generally recognise the importance of health records, and make statements like these:

> A health record shall be started and maintained for every person receiving health care services in a hospital, nursing home, community health centre or other health care facility.
>
> Health records must be kept confidential, current, accurate, complete and readily available for patient care.[2] ·

Making medical records is not just a responsibility of medical practitioners. Records are produced by different client care providers in different clinical settings. Yet, the basic requirements apply to all: entries must be legible and non-erasable, identified as relating to a particular person, organised sequentially in time, and made available to authorised persons. The accuracy and completeness of the records you make is relied on by others, and is an essential supplement, but not replacement, for a full verbal handover between staff.[3]

Taking notes and making records is one of the key skills of health professionals. It is vital in terms of effective teamwork. Other health carers dealing with that client need to know what has happened and need to be able to refer to detailed information about the client, without asking for the information all over again. (The delicate personal balance between disclosure and trust is explored further in the next chapter.) Concerns about privacy, and understanding when it is ethically acceptable to breach privacy, tend to focus on the notes taken by health care professionals.

There is a model of ethical decision making that has understanding the nature and extent of a medical condition at its centre. The model was proposed by Jonsen, Siegler, and Winslade. Their model has the following main elements: medical indications, preferences of clients, quality of life, and contextual features.[4]

You have treatment options available to you as a health care worker. Some of those options are predetermined for you, as discussed in Chapter 2. Some options are decided by the type or level of training and skill that you have achieved, as discussed in Chapter 1. Some are decided by you, using your considered professional judgement, in consultation with the client. The difference that social context makes to this consultation process, and the accompanying partnership between health care workers and clients, is receiving considerable attention from ethicists.[5] It is a delicate and complex relationship that requires an atmosphere of mutual respect and attention if it is to develop in a healthy way. The relationship is explored further later in this chapter, and in Chapter 4.

You read earlier that getting to know clients, at the same time as you begin to understand what has happened to them, is crucial. Unless you know a little about them, it may be difficult to respect and promote their autonomy. You might need to know whether when faced with difficult decisions, for instance, they would simply prefer to be left alone to think things through, or whether they would like to talk things over straight away. You might need to ask directly to find such things out, and you might need to undertake gentle questioning, or negotiating, to come to an understanding of what treatment or management plan the person would like or prefer (given a reasonable choice), and how they would like to receive it. Some standards of disclosure of treatment information rely on this mix of questioning and negotiating, as is discussed further on in this chapter, in the section 'Negotiating treatment'.

Exercise 3.3 Make a wish

We all have different thresholds in relation to being able to think about what we want, being able to express it, and being able to ask for something. We also have different thresholds as to how inclined we are to further other people's wishes. This is at the heart of who we are, and consequently, is crucial to how what we want might be achieved. This brief exercise illustrates how very different we are from each other.

In a group setting, ask the following question of the person sitting next to you: If you could wish for anything, what would you wish for? (Make it clear that you want them to tell you only one wish!) Make sure both of you get to tell each other your wish.

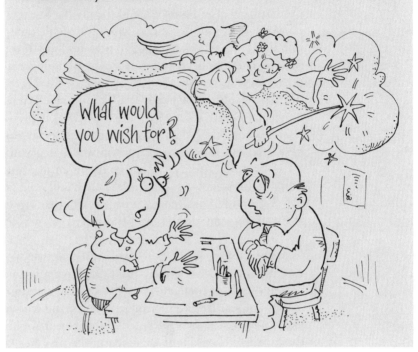

Whenever I have supervised this exercise I have noticed that a hush falls over the group, as people sigh, try to think of a wish, and then try to work out how to tell it. Some people have trouble thinking of a wish. Should you, if you believe in autonomy, help them to think about what they want? Or is it their right not to think of anything? If they have thought of something, but feel shy, should you help them to tell you? Or should you leave them be? (More discussion on privacy is included in Chapter 4.)

To return to the group exercise above, once the wish is expressed, group members should think about whether it is in their power to fully grant the wish they heard, or whether they could help the person part-way towards their wish. In other words, do they agree it is a good wish, and do they feel able or obliged to help? Ultimately, do they feel obliged to help the person in their pursuit of that wish? Their answers will indicate something about how much they value autonomy in its own right. To further autonomy as an absolute right is to further the client's wishes regardless of whether it would be the professional's preferred wish.

Some clients are risk takers, others are not. Cautious people might not want to go parachuting on their days off, but risk takers might. How people approach their everyday health, health risks, and treatment, when they become clients, varies in just the same way.

J. S. Mill, the famous early libertarian, thought that individual liberty should be allowed, within certain limits. This applied to the different liberties of consciousness, thought and feeling, expressing and publishing opinions, tastes and pursuits, and the liberty to unite with others for any purpose. The limits to liberty allowed by Mill were, broadly, serious and imminent harm, other's similar liberties, and threats to the fabric of society. These limits take into account the respect that we should afford others (as well as expect ourselves) and the need for all to live in a society that has established structures and boundaries. Interestingly, Mill did not think that liberty should be limited on the sole grounds that the person's choice would harm themselves. He thought that competent adults should be free to risk their own health and well-being without interference.[6]

We are used to limiting autonomy in an institutional context. If you think of our society, we have rules that tacitly limit autonomy on a number of grounds. For instance, a person who likes to drive will be allowed to do so, but only on the road. If the person likes to drive fast, we might say that that type of driving should be done on freeways, and not in suburban streets. Why? One explanation is that we have judged it too dangerous to others if these limits to driving are not imposed. So that person's wish or preference for fast driving should not be to the detriment of others. Another example is the person who likes to drive but also likes to drink. We say yes to each of that person's wishes, but stipulate that these things should not be undertaken together, as we judge drink-driving to be too dangerous to both the driver and others. Institutional bounds to autonomy and liberty are explored further in Chapter 7. Try answering the following questions. They will prompt you to reflect on the way you value autonomy, and how autonomy is limited or promoted.

Think of a situation in which it has been difficult for you to accept the autonomy of an individual patient or client. What did you do? Were you satisfied that you acted properly?

Now think of a situation in which the client's autonomy was limited, not by you but by the institution or resources. Were you satisfied that the principle of 'respect for persons' was upheld?

Now think of a situation in which you have promoted someone's autonomy. How did you do that? Were you satisfied that you acted properly?

The choices of an individual are made within a social context. Such decisions are therefore subject to social limits. Such limits are termed 'social morality limits'. Mill's essay 'On Liberty' suggests a difference between personal and social morality. That is, if something affects no other person, it should be in the realm of their own choice. However, if it affects others, by threatening the fabric of society, or by threatening other people, then it is a social issue, and the liberty can be legitimately constrained by social decision.[7] As a further exercise, you could make a list of what you think constitutes personal morality decisions, and what constitutes social morality decisions, in a health and medical context. You may like to consider the limits placed on the choices that an individual can make in relation to a public-health issue, such as smoking.

In our health care system, treatment choices made by clients are usually interpreted as questions of personal morality. In practice, we allow autonomy that is consistent with Mill's position. People can choose what type of treatment they would prefer, given a choice, and they can even choose not to be treated at all. Provided they are not harming other people too greatly, by for instance spreading an infectious disease, their choice about treatment is their own, and their reasons for making that decision must be respected.

One of the practical limitations of client choice is that such choices are often made within an institution. The institution may offer only a limited range of treatment options. In setting up institutions, we show our concern for the health of all people in society, and most limitations imposed by institutions are intended to protect the integrity and health of all people rather than any one individual. These limitations may be interpreted as social limitations protecting the social structure of the health care institution. For instance, under our health system, a public patient in hospital may not be able to choose their own doctor, while a private patient can. If individual public patients wanted to choose their own doctors, but could not pay for the doctors' services, we may feel justified in denying them that choice on the grounds that the system, as our society has set it up, can stretch to allowing them treatment options, but not their choice of doctor.

We may accept that it is more important to protect the social system than to promote autonomy. In Mill's terms, this means that we are prepared to limit personal choices in relation to the allocation of resources because the question is one of social morality. In a less strict sense, we have decided that people cannot have unlimited choice of health care and consequent unlimited spending on this health care because this would affect other people in society to an unacceptable degree.

The key to this is that autonomy and client preferences, or wishes, are not absolute. They must be weighed against competing liberties and interests. Professionals have their own threshold for allowing individual autonomy before they begin drawing boundaries to this autonomy. Philosophical stances can guide us as to when to place those bounds. Libertarianism is at one extreme, and even it acknowledges some limits on liberty. Paternalism is at the other extreme. And there are choices in between. These choices are set out in the section later in this chapter, 'Negotiating treatment'.

So far, we have established that what the person is like, what has happened to them, and what they would wish for or prefer, is ethically important. Their autonomy is important, but it is not absolute, and there may be circumstances in which you are not obliged to promote it, and even some circumstances when it should be curtailed. In any situation in which you are deciding to promote, allow, or limit autonomy, you need to consider the accepted standards relating to the extent of client choice. Sometimes there are clear standards to refer to, sometimes not. Legal and administrative limits can help, but as professional ethics is about reflection, these standards must always be assessed from an ethics stance as well. If you disagree with the standards on ethics grounds, you should challenge them.

Non-judgemental harm minimisation approaches are quite well accepted in health care when a patient poses a risk to him or herself, such as in illicit drug use. Gaining trust and understanding what substances are being taken is important, then different strategies can be used towards the goal of reducing use, while monitoring their health. One physician's advice is that in treating sports people who use performance enhancing drugs, the first step is encouraging disclosure of dangerous practices, and understanding why people choose to engage in them. If the sports people are elite and using drugs as a tool towards performance goals, they can be engaged but only over time. Recent gym users can be amenable to information about effective diet and training that can achieve the results hoped for more safely. For recreational users, other illicit drug use can be common, so different strategies may be needed. This physician acknowledges the illicit or dangerous drug use and works towards keeping each patient as safe as possible.[8] Can you work out which philosophical stance this harm minimisation practice is compatible with?

Different clients want different types of care. So do different subgroups in our society. You need to continually ask yourself whether you are equipped to provide the care they desire. The Western model of care, which attempts to maximise choice, views each adult as an individual agent, and has, as one of its aims, the prolonging of life, may not be culturally appropriate for some health care recipients. For instance, Qiu argues that Chinese culture reinforces group responsibility over individual choice; self-interest should not be pursued to the exclusion of the interest of one's family or community, and one's duties assume greater importance than one's rights. He notes that this communitarian approach does not occur so much in the West, where generally, an individualist approach prevails.[9]

These days, health professionals are trained to work in different contexts and to serve different cultures. You have the benefit of a more comprehensive knowledge of other cultures: by your ability to travel, live, and work in different countries, and by the fact that you live near a rich diversity of ethnic communities in your own home towns. So, you are partly prepared for the fact that people are different to you.

Yet we should still be aware that our culture shapes our expectations and understanding of illness, health, and care. Clients' expectations and understandings may be different to yours. Professionals' expectations should include getting to know the clients a little, understanding them for themselves, and beginning a health care relationship with them that is based on respect of their difference. Only then are you ready to take on some responsibility for caring for them.

THE BEGINNINGS OF TREATMENT RESPONSIBILITY

The decision to take on the responsibility of caring for someone under-pins health care. The responsibility to take on their care can be expressed as an obligation of doing good, also termed beneficence, as you will remember from Chapter 1. Beneficence is a tricky word, but its meaning is quite simple. It is pronounced a little like beneficial. Many students and professionals have trouble pronouncing it. Try saying beneficial a few times out loud, then change the 'ficial' bit to 'fecents', and put less emphasis on the middle of the word at 'f', and more on the 'n'. It is useful to remember that if something is beneficial for someone, it has often been brought about by an action that is beneficent.

You will also remember, from Chapter 2, that doing good can be defined in different ways by different professions, and that we may only be obliged to deliver that good if someone has a right to it under the model of justice that operates in our society or in our institution. Bear in mind though, that ethics is an ideal and optimal standard of behaviour, so even if there are constraints, it is plausible to aim to maximise what is regarded as good. The principle of beneficence implies an ideal level of care. It goes beyond what is accessible or affordable, or a just claim.

Consider this case from the UK. In the UK, there is ongoing reorganisation of aged care, including standards required of homes, public assistance for fees for residents, and allocation of subsidised care placements in designated homes. In this context, an elderly woman was required to move from the aged care home she had been in for some years. Cissy Townsend's doctor opposed her move from the care home, believing the 90-year-old's best interests were to remain in what she knew to be her home. Five days after the move, she sadly died, and the GP reportedly entered the cause of death as 'acute stress reaction to the move', refusing to list natural causes of old age on the death certificate. He championed her care, and continued to champion her interests in opposing the authorities' decision, despite the public interest in imposing financial constraints of public monies for each individual's care provision.

An inquiry ensued. The media coverage of the case extended over many months, and became a public petition for further government attention to the needs of old age pensioners, and specifically, individuals in aged care.[10] The commitment by the local doctor illustrates the nature of the strong responsibility the health professional feels to the individual patient. It is above the constraints of justice and resource allocation debates.

Exercise 3.4 Ideals of care

You could reflect on what sort of care you would like to provide, given an ideal environment for providing that care. Try completing the following statement.

In an ideal world, the sort of care I would provide is...

....

....

....

....

....

....

....

....

....

....

The heart of beneficence, of taking on a responsibility to care, is:
• the micro level of what is beneficial for the client
• the delivery of that benefit, or
• working towards that benefit in the context of the partnership between the health care worker and the client.

Health professionals routinely take on new patients or clients, or refer them on to others if they feel they either can't provide the care sought to the standard required, or can't provide as effective or timely care as another professional. The ethical issue is how hard you should try in providing care, and what care you should offer.

You also have a choice about whether or not to take on care; for example, whether or not to disclose your health care skills in everyday situations in which they may be called upon, and whether or not to disclose the extent of your capabilities in the course of caring for a client. On a group holiday, would you disclose that you are clinically trained?

Would you be prepared to adopt your professional role, if it could be helpful in the course of the trip (for example, for a broken arm or a serious allergic reaction)? Think about what you would be prepared and able to do in such situations. Of course, answering this depends on what resources you have around you, how serious the situation is, and who else is available to care. (Taking on treatment responsibility in emergency situations is also dealt with in Chapter 6.)

Once you settle on the scope of what you define as beneficent, you may be obliged to assist in that way. On a broad level, once you train as a health care professional, you may be obliged to use your training where your skills are needed. Clearly, the definition of beneficence has some force because it creates a responsibility. That responsibility can be interpreted as an obligation to assist and rescue whenever anyone is in need. The Australian philosopher Peter Singer believes that beneficence means that you must always act to prevent what is bad, unless something of comparable moral importance must be given up by performing the action—such as leaving yourself worse off than your potential clients. In Singer's framework other people's interests are equal to our own interests.[11] This is not quite a positive duty (an obligation to actively seek out ways of doing good), but it is a duty to intervene to prevent harm occurring. For example, if harm is about to be experienced by someone because of lack of food, shelter, or medical care, then preventing the consequent harm may require positive action, such as giving them some of your food, which could be said to imply some degree of self-sacrifice. Another example of this prioritisation of duty to others is the way in which religious orders and volunteers working in some countries place themselves in living conditions similar to their clients, and suffer great physical ordeals so that they can improve the lives of others. It often takes particular skill and special commitment to work in dangerous or exacting conditions. For instance, the rescue training for the ambulance service has been described as particularly 'physically and mentally demanding, very intense and demanding'.[12]

It is up to you to decide whether you think the level of service promoted by Singer is an obligation or a sacrifice. If you see it as a sacrifice, then you would view those who make this sacrifice as Samaritans. More importantly, not to do it would not reflect badly on you at all. The limits of a duty to care are more palatable to the professional if Singer's position is seen as a sacrifice, and this seems to be the professional consensus. For instance, few health care workers would see their responsibilities as extending to 24-hour vigilance, or treatment for all people in all parts of the country or world. Being a counsellor doesn't necessarily mean that you are obliged to work in crisis situations that you find too stressful. You can fulfil your obligations to beneficence by finding your own niche, and satisfying yourself that the work in crisis situations is being done by someone else.

Yet, this commitment is sometimes tested in your routine job, in unusual times of crisis.

Exercise 3.5 Duty and limits of care

As a group, work on the following scenario. The facts have been changed slightly from a real example from early 2003, when the SARS (severe acute respiratory syndrome) epidemic was reaching its peak. At the time, it was unclear whether the epidemic of the flu-like illness was peaking, but what was clear was that it was racing through many populations in Hong Kong and other areas of China, people had died in Singapore and Canada, and there were isolated cases in the USA and Europe. The sudden acute illness was affecting frontline health workers significantly, and schools were being closed, and sections of the community quarantined. Daily updates on numbers of people who had contracted suspected symptoms, as well as numbers of people who had died from suspected or confirmed SARS, were issued by the World Health Organization and local health authorities.

A local practice receptionist and health nurse, living and working in Hong Kong, with two young children, became worried that her work was becoming increasingly busy and demanding. She had seen her hours increase dramatically, as people flocked to the local doctor to have any symptoms checked, and ask about the symptoms of SARS. One of the practice doctors, an expatriate Australian, decided to take his family home, thus leaving fewer doctors and an increased workload for the practice. Those remaining were under stress, and were increasingly worried about their families if they should contract an illness from one of the patients coming to be checked. As the receptionist, she was the first to see any patients. She felt she had to make a decision whether or not to keep working, for her family's sake. What should she do? How could you advise her to go about making her decision? If she is a receptionist, does she have the same higher duties as a health professional? How far do those duties extend if she is practising as a nurse? And what do you say about the doctor who returned home?

Clearly, the extent of duties needs to be assessed by each person, given their own context, family responsibilities, and professional roles that they have undertaken.

It is not sufficient to just define beneficence and try to do good. Being a health care worker also carries with it an obligation not to cause harm. This is termed an obligation of non-maleficence. To be maleficent is to intend to harm, like the word malevolent. Health care workers must try not to cause harm. There is philosophical debate about whether actively causing harm, or allowing harm to occur through not intervening, is equally morally reprehensible.

Exercise 3.6 Responsibility for harms

Thinking about a scene from a murder–mystery novel by P. D. James may help you to decide if you think there is a moral distinction between acting and not acting, when harm seems to be the outcome of not acting.

In the scene, two children of about 11 and 9 years old are playing in the garden while their father clears out a part of the shrubbery. He is using a sharp bladed hook, called a billhook, to cut and pull the overgrowth away. Suddenly, the children hear him yell in pain and call for help. They both look from a distance and see him bleeding heavily, with a large gash on his thigh. The older child, a boy, drags his sister after him, but instead of pulling her towards their father, he pulls her out of sight and away into the orchard. She asks him to let her go so they can get help, but he holds her still against a tree. There they wait for a few minutes, until he releases her, and says that they can go now. When they reach their father he has died. The boy simply says that she has nothing to fear from now on.[13]

Try and list why you think each person, in this case children, is morally responsible for the harm or not, and why.

....

....

....

....

....

....

....

....

....

....

....

There are times when you, as a health care worker, have a choice about whether or not to act. You could, as an exercise, do a role-play of a health care situation in which there is a choice of acting or not acting, and demonstrate why you think each person in your role-play is, or is not, morally responsible.

'Smith and Jones' is a shorthand way of referring to a well-known scenario illustrating a particular type of philosophical conundrum: the moral import of acting or not acting; of killing or letting die. In one version of this scenario, a cousin (Smith) actively drowns his younger cousin (Jones); in the other, Jones watches and does nothing while Smith drowns. Inheritance is a key part of the scenario: in both versions, one person stands to gain from the other's misfortune. Rachels argues that the bare difference between killing and not killing is not, in itself, morally relevant.[14]

There are a number of philosophical doctrines to help us decide if harm is morally our responsibility, and to what extent that harm is our particular responsibility. One is the 'doctrine of double effect', which involves a distinction between what one foresees and what one intends. Harm may be morally forgivable if it is foreseen, but not if it is also intended.[15] For example, a psychologist who encourages a client to face their phobias, intending to, in the long-term, lessen their fears, may in fact cause the client to experience short-term anxiety. The psychologist can be forgiven if he or she has not intended to cause that anxiety, even if it was foreseen as part of the healing process. However, if the psychologist intended to cause anxiety for its own sake, he or she may be regarded as unethical because there was intention to cause harm.

The doctrine of double effect may also be used in more extreme cases; for example, a pregnant woman with a cancerous uterus may be told that, in the absence of intervention, there is a high likelihood that both she and her unborn child will die. The woman may decide to have a hysterectomy, and it would be an unintended, but foreseen, consequence that the unborn child would be aborted. Under the doctrine of double effect, it would be unethical if the bad effect (the abortion) were the means to the good effect (the curing of the cancer). It could not, however, be said of this situation that the abortion would be the means to the curing of the cancer. Rather, it would be the hysterectomy (in conjunction with further therapy) that promises to achieve that good effect. The doctrine of double effect attempts to achieve a balance between, on the one hand, the good pursued, and on the other, the harm that may accompany an attempt to do good. The action taken (in this case, the hysterectomy) must be good in itself, just as treating the woman for her cancer is good.

Some modern philosophers, such as Phillipa Foot, think that the crucial point is whether something is deliberately allowed, and this concept of deliberately allowing something encompasses both intended and foreseen consequences.[16] They would encourage us to acknowledge that harm from actions is often unavoidable, and they advocate weighing up the rights of the parties before deciding whether one is entitled to bring about some benefit for one person when another may be harmed.

Deciding what you can do as a health care worker depends on what can be achieved by what you can offer. The crucial test is whether it can bring about good, whether it really is beneficent. This decision as to whether or not it is good involves taking into account the other options available to the client. What you have to offer may not be appropriate. Jennett has provided a test (essentially rules of thumb) for deciding when a specific treatment is inappropriate. He proposes that if the treatment satisfies any of the following five criteria, then it should not be used:

1 It is unnecessary because the patient is not seriously enough affected to need it or the desired objective can be achieved by simpler means.

2 It would be unsuccessful because the patient has a condition too advanced to respond to or benefit from treatment.

3 It would be unsafe because the risks outweigh the probable benefits.

4 It would be unkind because the quality of life following the treatment is not likely to be good enough or long enough to justify such treatment.

5 It would be unwise because it would divert resources from activities that would benefit others to a greater extent.[17]

This test has been used not only in individual treatment decisions, but also in resource debates because it takes into account the good that may be achieved for one person, as well as the good that may be achieved through the same or other means for others.

Health carers assume that there is a right to receive treatment and that a comparison of rights and interests should be part of the decision. Because rights carry with them obligations on us to act, comparing rights is, in essence, a weighing up of our duties. Some rights are positive, and some are negative. Those that are positive oblige us to act in a certain way, and those that are negative oblige us to refrain from acting. The concept of rights and duties is also referred to in Chapter 2.

Beneficence is tied up with autonomy in that a client is free to choose a definition of good, is free to determine what an acceptable risk of harm is, and is free to make a choice between types of health professionals accordingly. For instance, someone who doesn't perceive mental health as part of their health would probably never go to a psychologist, and people who think that only active medical treatment can provide adequate physical care would not elect to go to a palliative care unit if they were diagnosed with a terminal illness (they would probably pursue active treatment as long as possible). So the client makes choices both within health care relationships and before even visiting a health professional. As the treatment responsibility is accepted and care begins, negotiation about the type of care begins, as does the real test of both the professional's responsibility to be beneficent and his or her commitment to autonomy.

A DYNAMIC RELATIONSHIP

There is a debate in ethics about which principle—autonomy or beneficence—should take priority. There is really only a need to consider this when these two principles come into conflict: when the professional definition of caring, and the client definition of what care they would like to receive diverge. Most beneficence models either give way to autonomy when the client's idea of good is very different to the professional's, or include autonomy as an integral part of the principle of beneficence.

If you were a paternalist, you would believe that your idea of good, and therefore, your interpretation of the principle of beneficence, was applicable to everyone. There would be no need to change your view on good or your interpretation of beneficence, no matter how different your client's views were to yours. That means beneficence could always override autonomy. In extreme paternalistic stances, there may be little need to ask clients for their consent before doing something that you believe is good for them, nor would there be a need to tell them all the options before asking them to agree to something that you think is good for them. Many people associate this with the old style of health care, particularly the old way of conducting medical practice.

The paternalism associated with medicine, as practised in the past, cannot be entirely attributed to professionals: patients also abrogated responsibility and autonomy. This attitude is captured in the phrase: 'Doctor knows best'. The move away from this position has involved a developing sense of shared responsibility and the development of the model of a dynamic relationship between health care worker and patient. The modern rejection of paternalism amounts to a belief that the patient has a responsibility to double-check that the good being aimed at by the professional is compatible with their definition of a good.

The model of beneficence that builds in autonomy still has something of that paternalistic attitude because it lets the professional define what the good is that they will offer. Ultimately, it is up to the client to make decisions within the limits set by the professionals, but the basic good that the professional is willing to help their client towards doesn't change. Pellegrino and Thomasma argue for 'autonomy within beneficence', as a model that is distinct from paternalism.[18] This model acknowledges the complexity of the illness of the client, as well as the professional input in determining what could be beneficent.

Many modern philosophers, such as Beauchamp and Childress, maintain that beneficence and autonomy are separate principles that can outweigh each other, but in different circumstances.[19] When they do depends to some extent on the type of decision being made and the broader philosophical framework you choose to work under. A dramatic example might be a person who is terminally ill, and who wants to be switched off life support. Autonomy may be upheld if that is done, but if you think that beneficence includes the concept of sanctity of life (regardless of quality of life), you may not be satisfied that turning off the life support is beneficent. If you are a deontologist, you will be less likely to switch off the life support because, under deontology, fundamental rules, such as observing sanctity of life, must be obeyed irrespective of the circumstances. If you were a utilitarian, on the other hand, you might decide that the present and future happiness of the person, their family, and even other members of society is best served by switching it off. So you solve the dilemma by placing autonomy above the importance of life preservation, and justify this prioritisation of values by arguing that, overall, everyone would be better off if the life support were to be turned off.

An alternative balance between autonomy and beneficence is found in the 'enhanced autonomy' model, which encourages both health worker and client to exchange views, information, and their respective understandings of that information. This raises the issue of the interpretation and value judgement of medical facts. If this is instituted solely by professionals it is paternalistic; the enhanced autonomy model has the client participating actively in the interpretation and judgement of medical facts.[20]

In some ways, adopting a framework that gives autonomy primacy challenges the role of the health professions in defining good at all. If there was perfect liberty, a client could decide what outcome they wanted, what process they wanted to achieve it, and could then seek out a health professional to deliver it.

Each treatment decision you make is tinged with this debate over defining care, doing good, and the extent to which the views of health care workers and clients should be taken into account in coming to decisions about treatment. The process of making treatment decisions is, therefore, dynamic. The same balance is not necessarily achieved in all decisions.

Exercise 3.7 Treatment process and decisions

In clinical situations, ethics issues centre on a real patient. Choose a case in which a decision of some sort needs to be made, and in which there are different views on what should be decided. If you or your fellow students have access to a clinical setting, try this exercise with the decision faced by a real patient, being careful not to identify the patient. You could also use a hypothetical patient, by constructing a case as a group. The discussion process has been suggested for a training program for nurses who train in a clinical setting.[21]

Gather as much information on the issue from the perspective of the patient and the family. Analyse and interpret this to help in defining the dilemma. Then list possible alternatives for actions, checking these with colleagues, supervisors, and a doctor on the team. Identify the most likely solution to the dilemma, and the advantages and disadvantages of each option. Try and keep your own views separate from the analysis of what the parties think.

In a clinical setting, the next step would be to consult each party to see if a consensual decision can be reached, or if there is one course of action with the most agreement.

Our cultural context is crucial in striking an acceptable (Western) balance between promoting client choice and choosing the best care on offer; in principlist terms, this is a balance between beneficence and autonomy. However, we should at least be aware that in some cultures striking this balance is not considered so important: doctors and health professionals simply do the best they can for the client, and the client makes very few real decisions about their own care. In some cultures, informed consent is not seriously pursued. It is not that health care workers are intentionally trying to limit autonomy or cause harm to clients, but simply that the health care workers do not think full information and choice will be most beneficial for the client. At a time of great vulnerability for patients, health professionals want most to care for the client; they want to take the burden of decision making so that the client can feel secure and gather their own resources for recovery. In some cultures, when a patient is terminally ill, professionals routinely would not disclose the prognosis, or even diagnosis, to the patient. This has been noted to be a feature of health care in some Asian countries such as Japan.[22] Health care professionals may, instead, inform the family so that the family can ensure that they can make the patient comfortable.[23] Patients in these cultures may appear to be less self-determining, and may be reluctant to decide anything in serious matters without consulting their family.[24]

That we, in Western health care, find lack of information and lack of choice for the patient unsatisfactory is a product of our preference for liberty. However, we would do well to remember that it was not all that long ago that our own patients were not told of their diagnosis of cancer at all, and even now, the process of preparing the client before disclosing the diagnosis can be fairly long-winded. It is not that professionals in other cultures are less committed to care, but rather that we, in Western health care, place a higher emphasis on autonomy, and have a different expression of caring.[25]

Our own emphasis on autonomy challenges our commitment to beneficence and non-maleficence. We must continually decide whether, as health professionals, we can collude in facilitation of harm if clients want something that we regard as harmful. We must decide whether allowing and promoting autonomy is a good in itself, along the lines of libertarianism, or whether the good we value is something more derived, like health.[26]

NEGOTIATING TREATMENT

Joint input is needed for treatment decisions to be made. The health care worker and the client exchange and discuss information. Each continually takes stock of the situation facing them. This is where good notes can be invaluable. The medical records serve as a record of what happened, what has been explored, and thoughts on what might be useful to pursue.

Information is so central to the assessment of condition and options that it assumes key ethical significance as well. Information disclosure on both sides becomes a key dynamic in negotiating treatment. The health care worker often holds significant pieces of health information as a result of their knowledge of health sciences, their ability to interpret test results, and their conversations with other health professionals.

Information disclosure from a health professional to a client is probably best understood in a consultation context. A role situation such as described by Beauchamp and Childress entitled 'Non disclosure of prostate cancer' is useful as a starting point.[27] In this situation a retired man has just had tests done as part of a routine physical work-up. His doctor knows that these indicate 'inoperable, incurable carcinoma'. The man has recently lost his wife, and is planning a trip to Australia. The man, as yet unaware of the test results, visits the doctor who says nothing of the indications. After he has left the doctor's office the man returns to ask: 'I don't have cancer, do I?' The doctor answers, 'You are as good as you were ten years ago'.

This type of scenario is essentially weak paternalism in action. The doctor's response to the man's question is not the only possible response. It was the response chosen by the professional, for the moment, perhaps to put off telling to a later date, perhaps because the professional wished to avoid imparting bad news. Telling bad news is part of health care, and it is dealt with in more detail in Chapter 4, in the section 'Veracity on both sides'. The essential part of the dilemma is that the doctor had access to information that could have affected a patient's decision about specific treatment or a management plan, or about their life. Should the practitioner have told the man about his condition when the man asked 'I don't have cancer, do I?'

Exercise 3.8 Standards of information disclosure

Three information disclosure standards have emerged in recent debates about disclosure in the health professions:
- **the professional practice standard**—information given to patients by professionals that is that normally disclosed to other patients, and as disclosed to other patients by peers undertaking similar procedures
- **the reasonable person standard**—information given to patients that a reasonable hypothetical person (in legal terms this person is referred to colloquially as 'the person on the Bondi tram', or in a British setting, 'the person on the Clapham omnibus') would want to know before consenting to the procedure
- **the subjective person standard**—information given to patients that is normally disclosed by the health professional, or reasonably desired by

the client, but tailored by the professional to suit the individual client's situation or specific concerns.

Returning to the Beauchamp and Childress scenario, in a tutorial situation divide into groups, with each group taking one of the three standards. Try to think of the response that the doctor would have given under each standard. Here are some ideas that other groups have come up with in the past. The 'professional practice' group often has the doctor talking to colleagues to hear their view on what to do. The central notion here is that peer practice in similar situations determines acceptable disclosure. The 'reasonable person' group often speaks in terms of what people usually want to know to make x, y, or z decision. A fairly common approach in disclosing information is then taken. The 'subjective person' group most often advocates entering into a conversation with the patient to find out whether he really wants to know (or if he is asking not to be told). If he does, the doctor then needs to find out how much he would want to know before disclosing further information. This group requires an atmosphere of negotiation between patient and doctor.

The information disclosure part of the consent process was dramatically re-examined in Australia by the High Court in the case of *Rogers v. Whitaker*.[28] The High Court found that the informed consent process in relation to a particular operation undergone by the plaintiff had been insufficient, and that all material risks, that were material to the patient, should have been disclosed.

Exercise 3.9 Administrative information and decisions

At some times of the year, wards have fewer beds available. Staff holidays are planned for, and fewer elective procedures are done over that time. There can be administrative decisions however, in units such as intensive care, that close beds for periods of time. This means that those beds are not available for critically ill people. Most critical care incidents are difficult to plan with any certainty, so the bed closures cause considerable concern. The availability of backup in intensive care units is relied on by clinicians when they undertake even routine operative procedures. This information of bed closures has an ethical dimension, and forms part of the background of material risks.

Consider an administrative decision to close one third of the twelve intensive care beds available in a tertiary care hospital over an upcoming holiday break. As a small group, discuss the ethical elements of that decision. Then decide: what information should be given to health care personnel working in the hospital, and what information should be passed on to acutely ill patients, and what information should be given to patients planning elective procedures.

In an ethics study on this topic, perceptions of clinicians and managers on the consequences of bed closure decisions were analysed. Concerns were raised over fairness, accountability of the decision, and poor prior publicity of the decisions to key staff.[29]

How much information clients should have before they make decisions depends on the philosophical framework that clients, carers, and our society are prepared to support. For instance, under a libertarian framework, in which each person decides what is best for them, and pursues their own best interests and happiness, the maximum information, and therefore, the maximum corresponding choice, would be available to them. Max Charlesworth writes that under a liberal society, restrictions on autonomy would be limited. Governments could still discourage excessive individualism, and could promote 'altruistic concern for others' and 'a recognition of community values', but the basic autonomous agent must have the opportunity to make real choices.[30] Under a paternalistic framework, on the other hand, lesser information and choice could be supported if such restriction was for the client's good. Strong paternalism, in which a client's expressed wish is overridden, is less common than weak paternalism, as Pellegrino and Thomasma write. Weak paternalism occurs when someone cannot give full informed consent or is not given full options, and the physician decides in advance what might be in their best interests. Limited or sole options that correspond with this are then presented.[31]

It is the reason for lack of full information disclosure that is ethically critical here. Time available in consultation, knowledge of medical jargon, and so on could be presented as reasons for presentation of limited information by a physician. Should any of these reasons be enough to impinge on the client's interest in full and informed consent? We could all reflect on why we presented fuller information for one client, or one procedure, and not for another.

While issues in health ethics are often 'considered in abstraction from the social and political context in which they arise', informed consent and the issue of information disclosure has succeeded in reuniting theory with practical context.[32] Informed consent and information disclosure is most usefully considered as a process that occurs in a social context; it is undertaken in the context of knowledge of acceptable political norms. Therefore, the best way to learn about it is not in textbooks, but in the everyday societal interaction and transaction. The exercise on informed consent that is in the next section highlights this everyday context.

SEEKING CONSENT

Informed consent is really a process, not a discrete event. It is a process of information exchange and autonomous decision making. The patient or client needs to understand the key issues in a proposed or sought treatment, and then, before that treatment is given, the client must have made an informed, voluntary, competent decision to go ahead with it. Patients often sign a consent form, but this signing is not, in itself, informed consent. It is merely one way of documenting a whole process. Particular issues involved in understanding information and competency are followed up in Chapter 5.

The responsibility for information disclosure falls largely to the health care worker. As the 'expert', the health care worker knows how to describe the process, and knows its risks and benefits (and their likelihood), as they are known to the profession. These risks should be communicated to the client so that a decision can be made about whether to go ahead with the treatment or management plan.

Some of the issues in information disclosure were addressed in the previous section of this chapter, 'Negotiating treatment'. This current section concentrates on the process of informed consent for procedures. (Note that in the health care context, the word 'procedure' has a particular meaning; it refers to intervention processes performed on patients by health care professionals.) However, not all the responsibility for information disclosure falls to the health care worker. Some information about the client's values, preferences, or wishes needs to be voiced also, as this may make a difference to the type or range of treatment offered. Ideally, this information should be voiced by the client.

Informed consent to medical treatment lies at the heart of concerns in ethics for client autonomy. Informed consent is about clients giving permission for examinations or procedures, with the optimal amount of information available to them. It is a health care quality issue that is being given increasing attention in health care contexts and in the training of health practitioners. Health students, medical students, and health practitioners can find the theory behind differing information disclosure standards difficult to grasp. The following exercise has been written with that in mind.

What do you consent to in your everyday context? You will find that the key feature of whatever situation you think of is that you seek something, or agree to something, and another person provides something to you. Write down everything you know about that process (and have experienced in it). Then, turn the tables: imagine that you are the one who is about to provide the service or process to others, and write a consent form explaining that process. The reality of health care is that health care workers provide something that others seek. Health care workers understand the process involved in the thing that is sought. Before they can provide it to others, who most probably have never experienced it before, they have to explain it in sufficient detail so that the potential patients or clients can decide whether or not to go ahead.

Exercise 3.10 Consent forms for everyday

Try writing a consent form for these everyday processes: having a haircut, getting your legs waxed, having your ears or other body part pierced, having a sandwich made, taking a bus ride, and going on a plane. You might like to think of others too. Before documenting the process and transforming it into a consent form that might be used for other people contemplating seeking these services for the first time, it is important to think about what you have experienced in these situations, and describe it in detail. Those contemplating engaging in these activities will want to know risks and benefits; likelihood of these; and perhaps, cost and future effects. The law terms this information 'reasonable knowledge of risks', and in ethics, it is said that to know such things is to 'maximise autonomy'. Providing such information is, in effect, enabling a full and informed choice.

When used in a class or group setting, the consent forms make for a lively tutorial-style discussion and some entertaining presentations when each form is read out. You will find that your colleagues are quite efficient at providing a range of information levels in relation to what the process or procedure would be like for the client, expected risks and benefits, and avenues for further information.

A consent form documents the patient's condition, the proposed or required treatment, the general nature and effect of the treatment, the significant risks or side effects of the treatment, reasonable alternatives and their risks, the views of the patient, how much the patient understands about the treatment, and whether he or she is able to consent.[33] There may be only a small space for writing these things down on the form. It is a shorthand document that points to a larger process.

Re-examination is a consistent theme in health ethics. In Australia, we continue to reflect on informed consent, with the NHMRC formulating guidelines on informed consent, to articulate current standards. The latest includes advice on how to allow patients to express their concerns, uninterrupted, how to deliver information to maximise comprehension of all risks, and how to allow further time for questions at the end of the consultation.[34] This is in keeping with prior advice that informed decisions rely on availability of full information about their condition, options, and risks and benefits of the different courses of action.[35] The process is perhaps more properly termed informed decision making than informed consent. In one landmark case, the High Court found that a surgeon breached his duty of care to Mrs Whitaker before operating on one of her eyes.[36] As a result of the operation Mrs Whitaker sustained a condition known as sympathetic ophthalmia, which rendered her almost completely blind. The surgeon did not provide Mrs Whitaker with full information about the procedure before he operated on her eyes. And specifically, he did not provide her with relevant information about the risks. This information would have allowed her to make an informed decision about whether to have the operation or not, keeping her own concerns and best interest uppermost in her mind.[37]

The court, expressing the standard expected by the community, emphasised autonomy more than many health care workers would. No longer is normal professional practice sufficient in the eyes of current law. Each professional in each clinical situation must ask themselves 'What further information is this client asking for?' Deciding this may be difficult, particularly as clients do not use the same language as trained professionals. They may not use the language of ethicists to say they want to maximise their autonomy. They may not use the language of health care workers to express their particular health concerns. Yet, even a hint of concern, or questioning in an indirect way, is now an indication that professionals should offer more information for clients to use in their decision making. This legal redefinition of acceptable standards illustrates how standards can change. It is perhaps not surprising that this judgment was handed down more than ten years after patients began to be called 'consumers' and began to be encouraged to become progressively more active in their own health care and health care decisions. Some assert that the level of information that needs to be provided is too high.[38]

After you have considered the standards for information disclosure expected in your context, you may wish to check whether the consent form you wrote as part of the earlier exercise:

- includes information on the processes involved in the everyday action you chose as the subject of the consent form
- includes information on the risks and benefits involved in taking that action
- includes options for further information.

Of course, a balance needs to be struck between informing a client, and overwhelming them. If there is too much information, they may not understand, or attend to, any more details on the proposed procedure or treatment processes. The challenge is to be able to communicate essential information, and have opportunities for more, and ensure that each client understands and remembers crucial pieces of information so that their decisions are informed. If minor risk or effects of small likelihood do not concern them in the slightest, then listing all of the effects may be more of a burden than a help in their informed decision. On the other hand, if the ethical significance of a process is important to them, such as the use of blood products in one part of a treatment (the religious significance of this is referred to in Chapter 7), then much more information may be needed. The ethical consequences, the social and personal significance, and the relevance of information are increasingly part of routine information disclosure in health care work.

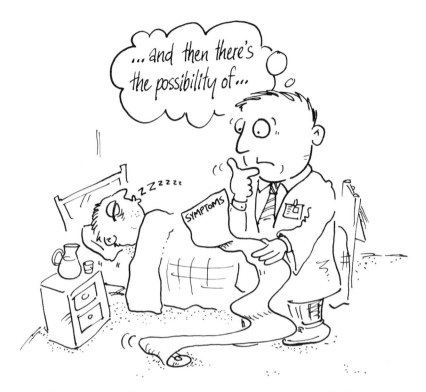

The key point is that you should try to look through the everyday nature of what you are doing when you provide a service. To people who are receiving it for the first time, it is not everyday. You need to take the time to consider what it is that you do, in an everyday sense, and then try to explain it to others and discuss what it means for them. After all, it is in the everyday that health professionals work. For you, as health care workers, a 'simple' operation is as straightforward as buying a sandwich or having a haircut. The challenge you face is to unpack the process and the things you take for granted about it; the process, risks, and benefits must be documented in minute detail so that they can be communicated and discussed with the health client.

Summary of key issues

- Respect
- Developing a relationship
- Being trusted
- Taking on responsibility
- Acting and not acting
- Taking notes
- Choice and autonomy
- Paternalism to liberalism
- Informed consent

Notes

1 P. Burnard, *Counselling Skills for Health Professionals*, 2nd edn, Chapman & Hall, London, 1994, pp. 96–7.

2 Audit Branch, New South Wales Department of Health, 'Health Records and Information', in *Patient Matters: Manual for Area Health Services and Public Hospitals*, New South Wales Department of Health, Sydney, June 1989 (updated regularly), section 9, policies 81/218.

3 E. O'Brien, 'Making a note and handover', Chapter 10 pp. 113–34, in C. Berglund and D. Saltman, *Communication for Health Care*, Oxford University Press, Melbourne, 2002.

4 A. R. Jonsen, M. Siegler, and W. J. Winslade, *Clinical Ethics: A Practical Approach to Ethical Decisions in Clinical Medicine*, 4th edn, McGraw Hill, New York, 1998.

5 J. M. Momber and R. M. Rueda, 'Bioethics and Medical Practice', *World Health*, 49th year, no. 5, 1996, pp. 29–31.

6 J. S. Mill, 'On Liberty', in *Three Essays*, Oxford University Press, London, 1975, pp. 92–114.

7 Mill, pp. 92–114.

8 R.T. Dawson, 'Drugs in sport—the role of the physician', *Journal of Endocrinology*, vol. 170, no. 1, 2001, pp. 55–61.

9 Qiu R-Z., 'Bioethics in an Asian Context', *World Health*, vol. 5, 1996, pp. 13–15.

10 McVeigh, A., 'Violet Townsend Inquiry Reaction', *The Citizen*, Tuesday July 22, 2003, pp. 12–13; 'We're improving our care services', *Gloucestershire Echo*, Tuesday July 29, 2003, p. 9.

11 P. Singer, *Practical Ethics*, Cambridge University Press, Cambridge, 1979, pp. 13–19.

12 Smith & Nephew Surgical, *Hospital and Health Services Year Book 1995/96*, 20th edn, Peter Isaacson Publications Pty Ltd, Prahran, Victoria, p. 34.

13 P. D. James, *Devices and Desires*, Penguin, London, 1989, pp. 92–3.

14 J. A. Rachels, 'Active and Passive Euthanasia', *New England Journal of Medicine*, vol. 5, 1975, pp. 39–45.

15 T. Honderich (ed.), *The Oxford Companion to Philosophy*, Oxford University Press, Oxford, 1995, pp. 204–5.

16 See, for example, Phillipa Foot, 'Killing and Letting Die', in J. L. Garfield and P. Henessey (eds), *Abortion: Moral and Legal Perspectives*, University of Massachusetts Press, Amherst, Massachusetts, 1985, pp. 177–85.

17 B. Jennett, 'Quality of care and cost containment in the U.S. and the U.K.', *Theoretical Medicine*, vol. 10, no. 3, 1989, pp. 207–15.

18 E. D. Pellegrino and D. C. Thomasma, *For the Patient's Good*, Oxford University Press, New York, 1988.

19 T. L. Beauchamp and J. F. Childress, *Principles of Biomedical Ethics*, 4th edn, Oxford University Press, New York, 1994.

20 T. E. Quill and H. Brody, 'Physician Recommendations and Patient Autonomy: Finding a Balance Between Physician Power and Patient Choice', *Annals of Internal Medicine*, vol. 125, no. 9, 1996, pp. 763–9.

21 D. Zeleznik, A. Habjanic, and D. M. Micetic Turk, 'Teaching ethics to students in the University College of Nursing Studies in Maribor', *Medicine and Law*, vol. 19, no. 3, 2000, pp. 433–9.

22 K. Hoshino, 'Information and Self-determination', *World Health*, vol. 5, 1996, p. 12.

23 D. Brahams, Right to know in Japan (letter), *Lancet*, vol. 2, 1989, p. 173.

24 Hoshino, p. 12.

25 C. A. Berglund, 'Bioethics: A Balancing of Concerns in Context', *Australian Health Review*, vol. 20, no. 1, 1997, pp. 43–52.

26 Max Charlesworth puts forward the libertarian position in M. Charlesworth, *Bioethics in a Liberal Society*, Cambridge University Press, Cambridge, 1993.

27 T. L. Beauchamp and J. F. Childress, *Principles of Biomedical Ethics*, 5th edn, Oxford University Press, New York, 2001, pp. 418–19.

28 *Rogers v. Whitaker* (1992) 175 *CLR* 479.

29 G. M. Rocker, D. J. Cook, D. K. Martin and P. A. Singer, 'Seasonal bed closures in an intensive care unit: a qualitative study', *Journal of Critical Care*, vol. 18, no. 1, 2003, pp. 25–30.

30 Charlesworth, pp. 3, 5, 6.

31 Pellegrino and Thomasma, p. 7.

32 The quoted text is from Charlesworth, p. 1.

33 Drawn from a sample consent form: Audit Branch, New South Wales Department of Health, no. 9.133.

34 NHMRC, Communicating with patients: advice for medical practitioners. Draft document, as at 2003.

35 L. Skene, 'What Should Doctors Tell Patients?', *Medical Journal of Australia*, vol. 159, 1993, pp. 367–8.

36 *Rogers v. Whitaker* (1992) 175 *CLR* 479.

37 R. C. Pincus, 'Has Informed Consent Finally Arrived in Australia?', *Medical Journal of Australia*, vol. 159, 1993, pp. 25–7.

38 P. Gerber, 'Has Informed Consent Become a Legal Nightmare?', *Medical Journal of Australia*, vol. 163, 1995, pp. 262–4.

4

The client and carer relationship

Overview

- Expectations and responsibilities
- Privacy and confidentiality
- Veracity on both sides
- Trust in the hands of the professional
- Risk to client or carer
- Risk to others
- Terminating a relationship

As the relationship of caring progresses, the expectations and obligations associated with it become increasingly defined. This chapter explores the boundaries of risk and the negotiated limits of care. Challenges to the relationship and different approaches to resolution are canvassed. The carer's broader responsibilities to others are discussed, particularly in relation to risk posed to others by clients or the treatment process. The expectation that carers will respond to this risk is also discussed.

EXPECTATIONS AND RESPONSIBILITIES

Clients expect to receive help when they are sick, and they expect to receive help so that they do not become sick. Our society is set up to provide this within reasonable limits, as discussed in Chapter 2, and some of you choose to become health care workers to provide this societal benefit of health care, as discussed in Chapter 1. When you become health care workers, others expect certain things of you, and you take on the responsibility of meeting those reasonable expectations.

In broad terms, we are all part of a reciprocity of interactions, expectations, and benefits. This reciprocity was explored by the philosopher

Hume. Hume made a distinction between natural virtue and artificial virtue. However, Hume's use of the word 'artificial' did not imply that he thought artificial virtues were not truly virtuous. He used the term 'artificial' to indicate actions that furthered the system of reciprocity that underpins society and aims to ensure the well-being of every individual.[1]

All members of society expect to receive the benefits that living in our society promises. As a health professional, you also play a role in delivering those benefits to others. Part of successfully delivering these is communicating clearly to clients what it is reasonable for them to expect, and what responsibility can be shouldered by the health professional.

Sometimes, clients seem to have wildly inconsistent notions of which treatments work, and which do not. What do you make of the following quote from a novel? 'His first heart attack had followed soon after, and Henry, half inclined to envisage his doctor as a personification of his illness, had declared himself much improved since the doctor had ceased to pay regular daily visits.'[2]

Some humour is being made of the patient's feeling that he gets sicker when the doctor comes. This is quite different from the doctor's own probable perception that the client gets well under his care (and then does not need further regular home visits). Checking perceptions and expectations every now and then might be useful.

You need to find a way to work together so that the expectations of clients and carers are similar and you understand each other's responsibilities. Professional responsibilities have been expressed, and are continually developing, in professional codes, as is discussed in Chapter 1. Patient responsibilities and expectations are now visible in patient codes, statements of patient rights, accreditation manuals, and patient handbooks.[3] There is increasing emphasis on the active obligation of clients to be part of the management plan, to take responsibility for attention to their treatment, and to take responsibility for their recovery and future health. The availability of information about professions and institutions may be crucial in forming appropriate client expectations.

Clients and health professionals engage in client–carer relationships with certain expectations of each other. One expectation held by carers, and addressed in Chapter 3, is that clients will trust you and will reveal their problem in detail, so that their care can progress. This disclosure on the part of the client requires them to trust the carer (this trust is discussed later in this chapter).

Within health care teams, different professions have different responsibilities. Each team member expects the others to work within their skill, with due care, and to shoulder their fair share of the responsibility in caring for the client. If something goes wrong, there is a team, as well as individual, responsibility to minimise the impact on the client. You need to check that each member is properly responsible and skilled.

Exercise 4.1 Accuracy and records

Think about the following example, which is from a Masters course in clinical ethics.

A nurse makes a mistake with the amount of medicine he dispenses to a patient. The mistake is realised by him and a fellow nurse. The patient's records show that the correct amount has been given. Neither corrects the records, nor reports the mistake to the charge nurse or the attending doctor.[4]

What do you think could be the effect of the mistake?

....

....

....

....

....

....

....

....

....

....

What responsibility is being degraded by not rectifying the records?

....

....

....

....

....

....

....

....

....

....

It is part of a health care worker's responsibility to be vigilant about and aware of the expectations placed on them and the responsibilities they bear in their professional role.

There are many opportunities for clarifying these responsibilities and for encouraging a team to live up to them. Generally, internal mechanisms have the potential to be educative, as discussed in Chapter 8.

PRIVACY AND CONFIDENTIALITY

You know you are in a private domain as health care workers because you hear personal details and see personal things that are not routinely disclosed or seen. You are in this privileged position so you can help. The initial disclosure of such information by clients is discussed in Chapter 3. Think back to Exercise 3.2 that asked you to disclose a secret to your classmate. Those people who chose not to tell their neighbours anything exercised their right to privacy, and we might think of those people as being inherently private. Those people who told a secret now have to trust that their neighbour will not tell anyone else, and that the confidentiality of that secret will be upheld.

We can and do choose to keep some secrets in our social interactions. Yet we also know that some information needs to be disclosed in the course of everyday life. We seem to accept that this is so in relation to dealings with many institutions, such as when we disclose details to our bank, to the taxation department, to our employers, and so on. Some health information needs to be disclosed for treatment to be decided on and provided. Some of this information is private, but that does not mean that clients need to tell everybody everything, or that health care workers should expect to know everything about their clients. You need to know as much as is necessary to provide care properly, and no more. Your respect for your client's individual integrity is demonstrated by allowing the client to make a decision about what is too private (or not necessary or acceptable) to disclose.

Whenever we have disclosed information that is private and personal, personal even if only because it has our name on it, we do so with an understanding of why it is asked for, and what it will be used for. Personal and private information includes verbal information, information about one's body, and disclosing one's body to view. It is when that personal information becomes potentially available to a wider audience that we become worried about privacy and confidentiality. We are worried because we have lost some control over how and what the information is used for.

Once information is potentially available to a broader audience, we further trust that those who seek access to it are authorised to have this access, and that they will respect it.

Exercise 4.2 Secrets and duties

Sometimes clients choose to limit how many people know about their medical condition, even when they are quite ill. Consider the following scenario:

An ambulance is called to a house where a woman in her late fifties has had a heart attack. Many of her relatives are over that day for a family gathering, and most of them are highly emotional about the situation and are unsure about what to do. The ambulance crew starts basic resuscitation measures, working through a routine protocol, when the local GP, who has also been called, comes rushing around the corner and says 'stop'. The family look totally startled, as do the ambulance crew.

Can you guess why the GP might have said 'stop'? Perhaps the GP knew something that the ambulance officers didn't, and even something that the family didn't know. What the GP knew was that the woman did not want active treatment in the event of a life-threatening situation. She did not want it because she wanted to die quickly rather than linger, and she was greatly influenced by the fact that she had terminal cancer, which she had not disclosed to her family. She had chosen to keep that a secret so that she could enjoy whatever time she had left without them worrying unduly about her. That was her choice, and as it happened, she suffered a heart attack prior to the expected onset of rapid deterioration in her health. The GP's knowledge of this was the reason he called out to the ambulance crew to stop active resuscitation. Unlike the family, the GP knew the woman's secret, and also knew her wishes. She was unable to inform the ambulance officers of her wishes because, by the time they had arrived, she was almost clinically dead. Whether the GP should have asked the ambulance officers to stop is addressed in Chapter 6, as is the question of when health care workers should stop active care. As will be discussed in Chapter 6, there is a difference between, on the one hand, care and comfort, and on the other, active restorative treatment.

Privacy and confidentiality are integral to maintaining human dignity and, as such, are concerns derived from the principle of 'respect for persons' (otherwise known as autonomy).[5] You may remember reading, in Chapter 3, about how respect for persons is essential in ethical dealings with clients and patients. The challenge in modern societies and health care institutions is to balance commitment to respect, privacy, and confidentiality, with the need for information about individuals.

The issue common to both privacy and confidentiality is respect for an individual's control over his or her personal information. Information privacy issues centre on control of access to personal information. Confidentiality issues are derived from privacy; confidentiality relates to control over the use or further disclosure of that information. In practice, privacy relates to what personal information should be collected or stored, while confidentiality is concerned with the storage, security, and use of personal data that has already been stored.[6] It is important to understand the difference between privacy and confidentiality because so many debates and guidelines draw the distinction. You may find the following explanation useful in understanding the difference.

Consider a 'private & confidential' notice on an envelope. The word 'private' implies that there is no public right of access to the information inside: only authorised persons should open the envelope and read its contents. To comply with this instruction is to recognise the interest that individuals have in being able to limit access to information; in other words, their rights to privacy. The word 'confidential' implies that those persons who are granted permission to read the contents have an obligation to guard against further lessening of individual privacy; for instance, by preventing non-authorised persons from reading the contents of the document. It also means that their use of the information should take into account its confidential nature: that its substance should not be revealed to others.[7]

This explanation illustrates the limited direct control that individuals have over their private information, beyond the initial disclosure. Individuals rely on their confidants to maintain desired levels of privacy and to use the information in the expected manner. They also rely on those who are not granted access to the information to respect that situation.

Think about what you might do if you had a letter delivered to you that was not for you. You could return it to the sender, or pass it on to the person who is the rightful recipient (if you knew that person) without opening it. To open the letter would be to pry. That feeling of prying is what you get when you invade someone's privacy. The rule that you should not open or read other people's private correspondence is fairly straightforward. However, you may receive correspondence where the name on the envelope is very similar to both your name and the name of your colleague. What would you do then? One solution would be to open the letter together, and together, read one line at a time until you identify whom it really belongs to. That way, neither person would read more private information than is absolutely necessary to identify the proper recipient.

Some simple safeguards in privacy and confidentiality can be undertaken at your work. Keep lockable filing cabinets locked, so that only authorised persons can open the cabinet and read files. If you are working with confidential material on your desk, cover it up when you have meetings with other people in your office. Other people do not routinely need to see the contents of all the confidential files in your office. And if you happen to be opposite someone else's desk and a confidential letter is in your line of vision, turn it over and say something like, 'I probably shouldn't see that and it is difficult not to notice it as I talk to you'. If you are discussing clients, you should do it in a private and secure area.

Next time you are in a public area, think about how common it is to hear sensitive information discussed by other people in places such as lifts, walkways, theatres, etc. It is amazing that such sensitive information is discussed loudly in public places; the participants in the conversation seem to be oblivious to the crowds of people around them, many of whom are only too pleased to have something to listen to as they wait for the lift to get to their floor, or for the concert to begin. It is a useful rule of thumb not to discuss work outside of work, and especially not to name patients or clients as you discuss their background or particular treatment scenario, unless of course, you are discussing the case with health workers who are part of the treatment team and need to know who the person is, and you are in a secure environment.

Within the work context also, there are things that constantly alert us to the presence of private and confidential information. When faxes are delivered, they are essentially opened letters. Only as much of the fax should be read as identifies the recipient; the fax should then be kept securely for that person. Some institutions use a folder, like a large envelope, so that faxes are not left for others to see, lying on desks or in pigeon-holes. Your institution may have different procedures for guarding privacy and confidentiality. Often, faxes have a special message printed on them, alerting us to the fact that they are private, in the same way that 'private and confidential' may be written on an envelope. To act on information contained in a fax destined for somebody else is a breach of respect. This, of course, also applies to the situation in which you hear private or confidential information that was not intended for your ears.

Institutions that routinely use fax machines balance the pressure for fast delivery of information against the risk to privacy and confidentiality. Safeguards are used, such as cover sheets, instructions on what to do if the wrong recipient receives the fax, and the practice of telephoning before faxing material (to make sure the recipient is standing by the fax machine ready to receive the fax). Here is one example of a printed message used on faxes to alert unintended recipients that they have duties of confidentiality.

This facsimile contains confidential information which is intended only for use by the addressee. If you have received this facsimile in error, you are advised that copying, distributing, disclosing, or otherwise acting in reliance upon this facsimile is strictly prohibited. If you are not the intended recipient, could you please notify us immediately.

Once information is disclosed, and once it is written down or distributed, we need to guard against lessening of privacy and confidentiality.

Some information needs to be written down in health care. Notes based on the information gathered about the client are called medical records, or health records. Those records are stored for further reference. As is discussed in this chapter, those notes should be accurate and complete so that they provide a good basis for following progress and making future treatment decisions. There is little ethical debate about that. It is when those notes are not safely stored, or when they are made available for a wider purpose than treatment of the individual, that ethics concerns are most prominent. The Medical Records Association of Australia, a professional body for medical records personnel, is acutely aware of this responsibility. In large institutions, organising files for easy access and protecting unauthorised access to files are the primary roles of medical records personnel. The code of ethics of the Medical Records Association states that members should: 'hold inviolate the privileged contents of the records under his or her custody or control and any other information of a confidential nature obtained in his or her official capacity, taking due account of statutes and of regulations and policies applicable to him or her or to his or her employer.'[8]

Exercise 4.3 Movement of information

Identify a piece of personal health information in your professional work and track its progress. Take a blank page and draw a box labelled 'information'. Draw a circle for each place that this information moved to, using arrows to denote the movement of the information. On your diagram, note who collected the information, who knows about it, who accessed it, and how it was used for the client's treatment. Then, look back through your trail and note the potential points at which information could be leaked or used for an unapproved purpose. Those leakage points may be at handover, at moments of minimal security, and so on.

You may also like to discuss if the following situation, or a similar one, would be likely to occur at your health care workplace. This vignette was written in a general-practice ethics project, in which general practitioners and consumers nominated their concerns and then met to discuss vignettes such as this one.[9]

A GP walked into the staff coffee room of his group-practice surgery and found the staff discussing (with a great deal of amusement) the diagnosis and circumstances of a patient of his who happened to be a well-known television personality. They were passing around a fax that had just been received with a report on the patient from a specialist consultant. The doctor remonstrated with his staff about confidentiality.

The real danger of each potential leakage point in the information trail you constructed for the last exercise is that while each person may genuinely need access to the information for the primary reason of client care, they may not understand the importance of privacy and confidentiality; in other words, they may not understand how important such ethical obligations are in a large institution, or society.

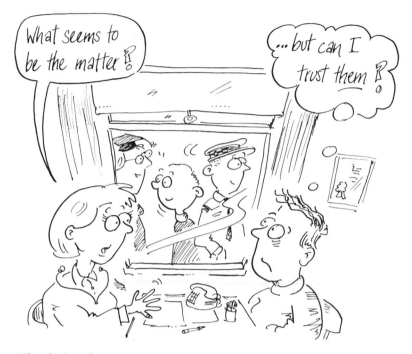

The lack of personal control over personal information, and the demand for this information by others, is of particular concern when information is collected in institutional settings, and when it is centralised and stored in computerised data banks. The danger is that if stored personal information can be used for another purpose, privacy interests will be overridden without adequate consideration of the importance of that further use, or in spite of professional concerns that confidentiality should be maintained.[10] A Swedish project linking 1500 individuals' medical, educational, and financial records, and an Iceland study holding detailed genetic information in a database are frequently cited as ethically problematic.[11] We rely on others, usually professionals or administrators, to use their discretion in deciding whether or not our information privacy interests should be overridden. In health care, clients rely on health care workers and records administrators to protect privacy interests and treat their personal information with respect.

Exercise 4.4 Regulated information

Different privacy protection applies in different contexts, but there is a trend in most jurisdictions to protect privacy of an individual's information, and improve security to ensure that. The information should not be transmitted further unless the individual consents to specific further use of the information, or there is explicit outweighing of public interests in that privacy to justify the transmission and use. In the USA, the professionals would need to keep in mind the Federal Regulations, and particularly the latest Department of Health and Human Services Privacy Rules, which came into effect in April 2003. They support patient privacy, in the context of sufficient flow of information for quality medical care. This regulation has had implications for the way organisations store their information, due to the security rules, and it has prompted the generation of standard consent forms for potential further use of the information, which practitioners can provide to the patient to sign if further use of the information is anticipated. It can be very difficult to recontact all patients at a later date to seek their permission, so it is sought upfront.

As an exercise in keeping up to date on regulations, try this internet exercise. You can generally get access to the internet at public libraries, if you do not have access at home or work or at a university. Look up the summary Privacy Rules, under the Department of Health and Human Services. For the web address, search under the department name, or go through the US government link. Then, look up one profession's response to the regulations. Journals such as *Nurse Practitioner* may be helpful, as practitioners share their views on how to comply with the regulations in professional practice.[12]

It is important to realise that individuals could suffer harm if a promise of confidentiality of personal information is not upheld. For example, if police were able to access research data that identified persons involved in criminal activities, those persons may be jailed. Embarrassment may also be caused by having clinical information disclosed in other contexts. This has been a feature of guidelines for modern research practice. In the 1970s in the USA, a number of Commissions into research participation collected instances of such embarrassing situations. The following extract is from the report of one of these commissions.

> As one witness told the Commission: ... a researcher was doing a follow-up study of people who had been enrolled in a methadone maintenance program ... The contractor had the name and address of one particular individual who had been enrolled in the program several years previously, and the contractor went to the individual's residence. It was a Saturday night and the person was having a party and the contractor said, 'Hi, I am so-and-so from such-and-such an organization, and we are doing a follow-up study of patients who had been enrolled in the methadone maintenance program.' Another such incident which came to the Commission's attention involved the recontact of patients who had received treatment at an abortion clinic. On both instances the recontacts were unwelcome, resented, and extremely embarrassing to the persons contacted.[13]

It is a separate philosophical decision whether such harm or embarrassment is justified, as will be discussed soon. The key point to note here is that there is potential harm in breach of confidentiality.

On a broader level, disclosure of information could also threaten the public's trust in the confidentiality of certain relationships such as banking, employment, and health care relationships. Health care relationships, in particular, are based on trust in confidentiality. A threat to an individual harms not only that person, but also others because it erodes their trust in similar relationships.[14] The essence of privacy and confidentiality is that information is disclosed under certain conditions; these conditions are particular promises of confidentiality and particular expectations as to how the information will be used. Truthful information is given in exchange for that trust. The professional's obligation to maintain the confidentiality of the information continues until the informants give consent to the further distribution of the information.[15]

The conflict is, however, that interests in privacy and confidentiality, just like interests in autonomy, are not absolute. The problem for all health care workers is in deciding when obligations to maintain privacy and confidentiality can be overridden by other obligations. These obligations can be overridden by competing interests.[16] The following are some examples of public interests:

- Society has an interest in the release of information that will assist in preventing other members of society from suffering harm. Societies need some personal information to assess the welfare of their members and to protect others from harm caused by infectious diseases.[17]
- Health care systems need access to personal information in order to assess their own effectiveness and efficiency and to improve so that others may be better served.[18] Access to information is justified if research is directed towards preventing harm to others in the future (this would be the kind of argument put forth by research organisations to support their access to information).

You can probably think of some more examples from other professional spheres.

There are some general rules for health care workers to consider in relation to the confidentiality of their health records or medical records:

- Confidentiality should be maintained, and consent sought for further use or disclosure of information, unless there is an overriding public interest. (This interest is generally mandated by another body, not just by the health care worker.) Thus, when public interest overrides the duty of confidentiality, it is legitimate to breach confidentiality. These interests include the reporting of infectious disease and the provision of evidence in criminal trials in response to a subpoena (and at the discretion of the court).
- Confidentiality should be maintained because otherwise there is the potential for harm to be done to the client, which would contravene the health care worker's duty of care to the client.

It is difficult to specify the precise circumstances that would justify infringement of privacy and confidentiality, apart from the sorts of extreme public interest provisions mentioned above. The primary question in relation to the release of information in the ordinary course of health care is 'Does the information disclosure serve the purpose of the treatment that the patient originally agreed to?'

Whenever there is a request for information disclosure, professionals need to identify the full extent of their obligations to both keep information confidential, and to disclose it. Consideration of the distinction between public and private interests may be a useful part of this process of identifying the extent of obligations.

The distinction between public and private interests in privacy is similar to Mill's distinction between social and personal morality, which was discussed in Chapter 3. Generally, public interests affect groups of people as a whole, whereas individual interests affect individuals in particular circumstances. Individual interests in privacy are generally upheld, except where there is a substantially greater public interest that cannot be achieved if that private interest in privacy is allowed. An example of a public interest in privacy is the need for trust to be maintained in confidential health care relationships so that members of society are not dissuaded from seeking health care for fear that the information they give to health carers will be disclosed to all and sundry. This is a public interest because this safeguard is needed to maintain a healthy society. An example of a private interest is the need for information to be guarded carefully because individuals may be harmed, socially, if their information is disclosed.

J. S. Mill said:

> ...as soon as any person's conduct affects prejudicially the interests of others, society has jurisdiction over it, and the question whether the general welfare will or will not be promoted by interfering with it, becomes open to discussion. But there is no room for entertaining any such question when a person's conduct affects the interests of no persons besides himself, or need not affect them unless they like (all the persons concerned being of full age, and the ordinary amount of understanding). In all such cases there should be perfect freedom, legal and social, to do the action and stand the consequences.[19]

The codes of ethics of health care professionals generally offer the advice that privacy is not absolute and can be overridden. (See, for example, clause 1.1.(l) of the Australian Medical Association's Code of Ethics, which states that such circumstances are when there is 'serious risk to the patient, or another person', as required by law, or as part of approved research, or 'where there are overwhelming societal interests'.)[20] The codes often have little practical help about which interest should take precedence.[21] This means that further professional discussion is essential. From time to time, when professional codes explicitly acknowledge this conflict and admit that the right of privacy is not absolute, there is controversy. Under the Australian *Commonwealth Privacy Act 1988* consent for further use of information is affirmed as the essential safeguard of privacy.[22] This Act originally was limited to Commonwealth agents and agencies, such as Commonwealth health institutions, but was extended to the private sector by the *Privacy Amendment (Private Sector) Act 2000*. They provide a number of information privacy principles that guide collection, use, storage, and further disclosure of personal information. The requirement for consent for that collection, use, storage, and further disclosure can be waived when disclosure, or use, fulfils one or more of the following conditions:

- it will 'prevent or lessen a serious and imminent threat to the life or health of the individual concerned or another person'
- it is required or authorised under law
- it is necessary for the enforcement of a criminal law (or the payment of a penalty in the criminal justice system)
- it is to protect the public revenue, and
- it is directly related to the initial purpose for which the information was obtained.[23]

This acknowledges the competing interests to privacy interests. Some public interests rely on the flow of information, such as in human rights protection and for social interests, and for business interests. This is a legal example of social limitations in action. Individual liberty and, in this case, privacy are supported, but limits are placed on both by public concerns over the welfare of other members of society, and over the strength of the fabric of society.

In the case of health research, there are NHMRC guidelines and discussion papers about the balance between the public interest in access and the public interest in privacy (NHMRC discussion), and under the *Privacy Act*, the use of personal data for research may constitute a specific exception to the general requirement for a consent process.[24] However, only ethics committees are in a position to decide this, and they must be satisfied that the public interest in the promotion of the research 'outweighs to a substantial degree the public interest in adhering to that Information Privacy Principle'. The guidelines and ethics committee application of them were thought to be operating well in late 2003.[25] Generally, people other than the health care worker make the judgement as to whether one public interest outweighs another. The health care worker still needs to consider any request for confidential information and should refer it to the appropriate authorities if the request is clearly not consistent with the purpose of treatment. This judgement as to the relative merits of different interests is tested in court from time to time. For instance, in 1992 a court was asked to decide if the Red Cross should be granted immunity from disclosing the identities of blood donors to persons subsequently infected by blood donation. The court considered survey results (the survey having been done for the court hearing) that showed that many people would not donate blood without confidentiality assurances. The court ruled that the public interest in assuring confidentiality, so that people would continue to donate blood, outweighed the interests that those infected had in disclosure of the identities of blood donors.[26]

When health issues pose a risk to others, the information can become 'notifiable', which means that it is mandatory to release to a relevant public authority. The severe acute respiratory syndrome (SARS), which began in November 2002 and reached the most serious epidemic proportions in China by mid 2003, was legislated as a notifiable condition in many countries. Quarantine provisions, that is limiting movement of people affected, or people in contact with those affected, were also made on public interest grounds. The World Health Organization requested countries' cooperation and central reporting of SARS cases and infection patterns, and health outcomes were routinely available on a public website, as soon as they became available to WHO.[27] WHO also became involved in issuing descriptions of symptoms to be vigilant for, travel warnings, and containment advice, as it tracked the epidemic in countries worldwide. In ethics terms, the measures were justified on grounds of serious and imminent risk if the information was to remain private.

Exercise 4.5 Organisational regulation

As a tutorial exercise, find out what one organisation's policy was on SARS. You could try your university, workplace, or local school as examples. See if there were travel restrictions, or limitations on attendance after travel, or exclusion based on symptoms, and so on. Find out how the policy was argued in terms of ethics, and take particular note of any wording on risk and interests.

If you had an opportunity to rewrite a policy, what would you suggest? Take into account the symptoms and health consequences (including the mortality and spread of SARS). You will find crucial facts to consider on the WHO website at <www.who.int>, or in local health warning documents.

It is likely that we will always have to live and work with the reality of both the duty of confidentiality and the demand for access to health care information. This will continue to pose challenges, with rapidly developing technology, communication over great distances, and the ever-growing networks of health care workers involved in the care of individual clients.

VERACITY ON BOTH SIDES

In a treatment relationship there will be points of progress and points of decline. There will be good news to tell in relation to progress, and bad news to tell if prognosis, or diagnosis, is grim or is not what was hoped for. Some health care workers are better at being frank with their clients than others, and some clients are better at hearing the truth than others. The willingness to relay bad news, for instance to discuss imminent death with a client, and the emotional preparation for it, is increasingly regarded as part of professional skill. If you choose to have an open and frank relationship with your client (and this is a culturally influenced decision, as is discussed in Chapter 3), you are upholding veracity. Upholding veracity does not necessarily mean telling a client all the bad news in one sitting. When the results of HIV test-results or cancer results become available it is common to have a number of meetings with the client so that the information and its implications can be discussed, and future management can be planned, as the client gradually comes to terms with the bad news.

Breaking bad news was the subject of a vignette in Chapter 3. Any bad news told to a client needs to be relevant to the client and must be information that is used in the further treatment or management of the client's condition. How risk or information is told can dramatically alter the dynamics of the client's recovery process. It is important not to destroy a client's hope, as hope is essential for recovery and for achieving the best quality of life possible.[28]

There is some concern that professionals are not trained to uphold veracity, or be truthful, with sufficient vigour. This has been noted particularly in competitive training settings, such as medical school. While senior researchers have, with some surprise, discovered instances of cheating and lying by students, students themselves do not register the same level of surprise at these findings.[29] Students report doing what they can to get through.

In her prize-winning essay on ethics, medical student Tara Young reflects on the way in which some of her fellow students lied and presented a false picture of their ambitions when trying to secure training placements in particular fields of medical practice. She observes the discrepancy between this behaviour and the centrality, to medicine, of honesty in dealings with colleagues and patients, quoting the American Medical Association's code of ethics: 'a physician shall deal honestly with patients and colleagues, and strive to expose those physicians deficient in character or competence, or who engage in fraud or deception'. Veracity with colleagues and clients is part of the trust-forming relationship between society and professionals and between individual practitioners and their clients.

People are increasingly asking how, if we condone (or even encourage) degrading of veracity with each other (in our personal and professional lives), we can uphold veracity with our clients. There is now attention being given to reinforcing veracity in all dealings between those involved in health care—students, professional peers, educators, clients, and the general public—as a first step towards veracity in health care relationships. In the context of health care education, we should encourage students to say if they don't know something, rather than having them pretend that they know (and try to bluff). There is a danger, as there is for all professionals, that in pretending to know something, you may overstep the bounds of your own skill, and make a mistake: a client may be given the wrong information, or a procedure may be conducted incorrectly. It is ethically responsible to acknowledge that you don't know something. Such an acknowledgment is an active reflection on the limits of your skill, similar to the skill-limit exercise you did in Chapter 1. When this happens it is your professional responsibility to remedy the deficit in your knowledge, to apply your newfound knowledge to the problem at hand, and to implement proper treatment once you know what to do. In short, it is acceptable to not know, and to admit it; but having done so, it would be ethically irresponsible if you then failed to remedy the gap in your knowledge or skill.

The previous chapter focuses on consent and disclosure of important information by the professional to the client. Some of the information disclosed could be test results, some could be the client's physical status, and some could be what treatment options were available, and their concomitant risks and benefits. Recently, ethics and law has also focused on whether clients are entitled to see their own medical records for themselves, and whether they have a right to access those records. It is generally acknowledged that the client does not 'own' the record, as it was made in the course of treatment, by a professional, for the purposes of professional assessment and management. The record includes 'aides de memoires' (French for memory aids or triggers), as well as personal information about the patient. Yet, as it is primarily about the patient, shouldn't the client be able to see it? Shouldn't there be frankness and veracity about its contents?

This was tested in the Australian court case *Breen v. Williams*, which went to the High Court.[30] In the judgment the High Court found that previous cases did not provide them with a basis to enforce a right of access, although it was suggested that this was now in the province of those making laws (politicians and drafters of legislation).

There is concern that some information could be harmful or distressing to clients, and that the information should only be available if professional explanation and counselling are also available. This concern amounts to a belief that any disclosure of information in medical records should really be done in the context of normal consultative disclosure processes, and is less about veracity than about healthy and full communication between practitioner and client.

TRUST IN THE HANDS OF THE PROFESSIONAL

Clients have significant trust in their carers. Whatever process or procedure you are undertaking with your patients or clients, you can probably sense that they trust you are doing the best you can for them.

Professional standards bodies, and ethics committees, are worried if the trust that clients have placed in their carer is abused. The abuse of trust is taken seriously because it goes to the heart of health care. When they need help, people are vulnerable, exposed, and dependent. If their trust in their carer is threatened, they may feel unable to return to the health care situation, even when they need care.

The general public should also be able to trust that decent care will be available to them. Stories of abuse of trust can have a lasting impact on the trust that a community has in a professional, a profession, or an institution. One example of the trust placed by the public in health care workers is trust in maintenance of confidentiality, which is discussed above.

In the late 1990s, a Victorian health care worker was barred from practising medicine because he was found to have breached, on a number of levels, both professional standards and the trust placed in him as a health care professional. The *Daily Telegraph* newspaper reported: 'He has been found guilty of abuse of trust by having sexual intercourse with two current patients, by flagrantly defrauding Medicare, by misusing the doctor–patient relationship to borrow large sums of money from existing patients'.[31] The basis of trust was abused in a number of ways. Even just one of the abuses could have severely damaged the basis of trust. The issue of sex between practitioner and client has received significant attention in the press, and before professional standards bodies, because of its potential for extreme damage to the trust and care involved in the relationship between provider and recipient, as well as its potential to deter other members of the community from seeking help because of fears that the same could happen to them.

On a different level, a hypothetical story of potential abuse of trust in the context of a, seemingly routine, first procedure conducted by health care students has been published in the *Canadian Medical Association Journal*. (The essay, by Caroline Shooner, came second to the essay by Tara Young, which was noted above.) The patient in the story, John Brown, is to have a chest tube inserted, and the resident invites the third-year (post-graduate) medical student to perform the procedure. When they go into the patient's room, her anxious expression, slight hand tremor, and sweating is observed by the patient, who asks if she has inserted chest tubes before. The resident replies: 'Don't worry Mr Brown, Jane is familiar with this procedure. I myself have done it many times. We are going to perform it together. Everything will go fine.'

Shooner points out the possibility that the patient has lost trust that capable and experienced medical staff are handling his care, and also that he has agreed to the type and manner of performance of procedures. In other words, the patient's belief that the doctor has been honest and comprehensive about disclosing the particulars of his treatment has been shaken. In this story, the moment of loss of trust passes, thankfully, as the procedure is performed skilfully, and the student is congratulated on the skill she showed.[32] Nevertheless, the potential for loss of trust challenges the way students are used in real health care throughout their training. It is usually seen as an issue of truth and veracity that students divulge that they are trainees and disclose their level of skill with the planned procedure. There simply has to be a first time for every procedure.

You may like to think back to the first time you performed a certain process or procedure. Do you think you had the trust of your client? Do you think you deserved that trust?

RISK TO CLIENT OR CARER

Health care is, by its very nature, a risky business. You, as a health care worker, will be in contact with people who are ill, or injured, or both. You will be exposed, sometimes, to dangerous situations and you will also expose your clients to some risk. Actively doing good and intervening often entails some risk. Your skill and care can minimise that risk. Institutional factors also influence how risky a procedure may be.

The following exercise explores one type of risk in the health care situation, and asks whether a proposed way of dealing with that risk can be seen as ethical. The risk is HIV transmission in health care situations, either from patients or from professionals. The proposed way of dealing with that risk is mandatory HIV testing of patients and professionals. You will have seen this issue aired in the media and no doubt in your professional circles. This exercise gives you a chance to try out some of the arguments for and against mandatory HIV testing. It has been written up more fully as a teaching exercise in the journal *Medical Education*, and if you are undertaking this as part of a class or with colleagues, you may wish to refer to the full paper.[33] This exercise presents a contemporary dilemma that invites discussion of philosophical theory and ethical principles. There is no one answer to the exercise. It is designed to elicit opposing answers so that you learn about ethics as something that emerges from the construction of an argument. If you have a couple of groups working on different arguments this exercise will take about one hour.

Exercise 4.6 Mandatory information gathering

Undergraduate and postgraduate health students are training in the age of AIDS. They are likely to work with HIV (human immunodeficiency virus) and AIDS (acquired immunodeficiency syndrome), a disease which, now twenty years after first being identified in the early 80s, continues to evade researchers and clinicians. It is a long-term disease that poses serious and life-threatening risks to sufferers.[34]

Understandably, health carers and health care institutions are concerned about HIV/AIDS issues. The majority of Australian institutions surveyed in 1991 listed treatment of HIV and AIDS patients as an ethical concern, second only to the issue of 'not for resuscitation' orders.[35] The concern centres on the fact that HIV is a blood-borne virus. Exposure to blood or other bodily fluids that contain the virus could pose a risk to others. Transmission could occur from patients to other patients or professionals, or from professionals to patients. Fear of contagion is a primary concern of health professionals dealing with AIDS, as evidenced by a Canadian survey.[36] Internationally, there has been extensive ethical debate over whether health carers are obliged to care for people with HIV or AIDS, given the potential risk to their own health.[37]

Patients with HIV/AIDS undergo numerous invasive procedures in the course of the disease, from repeated blood tests to more invasive procedures such as biopsies. It is arguably the more routine bedside procedures that pose the greatest risk of transmission from patient to professional. In the course of the procedure, the professional may prick himself or herself with an instrument that has been used on a patient.[38] Needlestick injury appears to be very common. One survey found that, over a two-year period, all surgeons and roughly half of the medical-unit doctors, ward nurses, and emergency staff in a major teaching hospital in Australia had 'stuck' themselves at least once. Students also reported that they had been 'stuck'.[39] Workers not in direct contact with patients, such as laboratory staff or cleaners, are also at risk of occupational exposure.[40]

It is estimated that needlestick injury with HIV infected 'sharps' carries a 0.4 per cent risk of HIV transmission and development of HIV antibodies.[41] This is a small but grave risk, given the potential seriousness of the disease.[42] Minor-surgery situations have alerted physicians and patients to the risk of transmission from patient to patient.[43]

The HIV status of professionals is also under scrutiny, although no risk of transmission has been calculated. Situations involving dentists and doctors with surgical duties have received greatest prominence.[44] The suggestion is that the likelihood of transmission from a professional is greatest in invasive procedures, when there is considerable exposure to blood and therefore possible transmission to the patient.

Such concerns about possible transmission have led to calls for mandatory HIV testing of patients and professionals.[45] These calls find some support in position, and policy, papers advocating that while autonomy and testing should only occur with consent, there should be exceptions if there is 'serious and imminent risk' to others, or if testing is thought to be necessary for 'clinical management purposes'.[46] Whether such exceptions are justified is hotly debated. Many commentators have argued that protecting the rights of persons with HIV/AIDS should take precedence.[47] There is no conclusive evidence that 'knowing' a patient's HIV status reduces the risk of needlestick to a professional. The use, by professionals, of 'Universal Precautions' (the term used for accepted infection-control standards) and routine hygiene, such as handwashing between patients to prevent any cross-infection (even in the absence of knowledge of any viruses), is under scrutiny.

This situation poses an ideal dilemma for ethical discussion, enabling both health care workers and students to learn about ethics as a tool for structured and rigorous debate where complex and emotive issues are concerned.

From what you have just read, try constructing a few points in the arguments for and against mandatory HIV testing. You could take as a starting point the writings of J. S. Mill, which are about the philosophical importance of liberty and of not putting others at risk. Mill described different types of liberties, of thought and action, and claimed that all people had a right to exercise these as they wished, and should only be 'interfered' with if others were at risk. 'The only part of the conduct of any one, for which he is amenable to society, is that which concerns others. In the part which merely concerns himself, his independence is, of right, absolute. Over himself, over his own body and mind, the individual is sovereign.'[48]

The four possible positions in the arguments for and against mandatory HIV testing for professionals and patients are represented by the quadrants in the grid, which you could make use of in noting your points. The arguments about this really hinge on the definition and perception of harm and of risk of that harm. It is quite appropriate that the expected risk of harm is lower for professional-to-patient transmission than it is for patient-to-professional or patient-to-patient transmission. That is because any 'sharp' that has the blood of a professional on it should be immediately discarded and should not be near a patient. That is in contrast to a sharp with the blood of a patient on it, which is routinely discarded by the health professional, before or during which time the professional may 'stick' himself or herself. There are high-risk situations in which professional injuries may occur while the professional is in contact with the blood or fluids of the patient, most commonly in surgery.

The exercise also prompts assessment of the relationship between the particular liberty and the particular harm. For instance, it may be that what is required is improvement of the universal precautions to prevent cross-infection, rather than knowledge of the HIV status of a patient or professional. This exercise illustrates that in order to construct arguments about ethics, it is necessary to have a good grasp of the facts (in this case, clear information on risk and on the benefits of mandatory testing). Ethical arguments are perhaps best constructed in conjunction with fellow professionals who can provide this crucial factual information.

After you have completed your basic grid arguments, you may feel you want to apply the reasoning to specific vignettes.

On the same theme, you may also like to consider the following hypothetical vignettes.

A young man comes to your practice or hospital for treatment. He has injured his leg in a car accident. Conscious and alert, he tells you that he is HIV positive. He is bleeding profusely, and requires treatment to stem the flow and repair the limb.

MANDATORY HIV TEST: ARGUMENT GRID

	mandatory testing	no testing
patients		
professionals		

You might like to think about how you would have reacted ten years ago, and how you would react now.

And another hypothetical vignette:

A patient is to undergo elective surgery, which you will perform. She notices that you have recently injured your hand, which has been sutured, but also that the injury has not yet completely healed. She asks that you undergo a blood test for HIV, and that she be told the results before the operation.

Consider how you would feel about the request, and what you think you should do, in relation to both your wound, and the requested test.

These vignettes raise issues of infection control, and patient and carer risks and responsibilities. They also raise the ethically perplexing decision of whether health carers who have ethical objections to a particular form of treatment (or some other aspect of the client–carer relationship) have an obligation to take on the patient concerned and be responsible for treatment. You can use these vignettes to ponder on privacy and secrecy, and to consider whether there is any difference between risks posed by clients to carers, and risks posed by carers to clients. The issue of privacy is dealt with in more detail in Chapter 3. You could use the same series of exercises with hepatitis C, which is also a serious virus, transmitted by blood contact, such as in reused intravenous equipment. Liver failure can result from hepatitis C infection.

RISK TO OTHERS

Posing risk to others is, in essence, a public-health risk. Debate can centre on whether there actually is a risk, and in what circumstances. HIV/AIDS, for instance, is a blood-borne issue, and it is dubious whether it should be described and treated as a significant health risk (contagion in the course of normal population contact, such as airborne contact). Tuberculosis, on the other hand, is clearly a significant public-health risk, as it is airborne. This assessment of risk is crucial. Unless the level of risk is established, infringement on one person's rights in the interests of the rights of others is very difficult to justify ethically.

In Chapter 3, you read that caring for the client and for others is an important feature of the health care worker's duty to care. Chapter 3 explores confidentiality and trust in a professional caring relationship, as examples of aspects of this duty. It discusses the fact that while the duty to maintain confidentiality is strong, it is not absolute: it can be breached where risk to others is involved. In some situations of significant and imminent risk of serious danger, there can even be a duty to disclose confidential information. This duty was tested in the famous legal case *Tarasoff v. Regents of University of California*, in which a patient told a psychiatrist that he (the patient) was planning to harm someone. The psychiatrist was found to have a duty to disclose so that the person the patient was planning to harm could be protected.[49] This duty was said to depend on whether the potential victims are identifiable and whether other protective mechanisms are available.[50]

The client can act to minimise risk to others. For instance, after a person gives blood to a blood bank, their blood is tested for a range of hepatitis conditions. If there are positive results for any of these conditions, the patient is informed and counselled to pursue health care for their own benefit, and they are advised on behaviours that pose risk to others. Their blood is discarded from the donor pool. There is a large degree of trust placed in the individual to minimise their risk to others so that the infection can be contained.

Quarantine wards attempt to balance the aim of treatment with the aim of protecting others in society from diseases. Looking back into the history of quarantine we can see that there are instances where it has been applied too widely—for instance, the practice of isolating people with developmental or mental disabilities. The balance (between treatment and protection) of risk that society is prepared to accept determines the laws and regulations that health care workers then implement. Further discussion on community input into deciding acceptable risks and benefits is included in Chapter 7.

TERMINATING A RELATIONSHIP

The ending of a health care relationship is a natural consequence of the beginning of that relationship. While the process of ending a health care relationship is studied by many, such as rehabilitation workers, acute care workers, and counsellors, it is sadly neglected by others.[51]

Once a task has been completed and the objectives of the relationship have been met, it may be time to move on to a new set of objectives. There can, of course, be reference points for reassessment. Your level of satisfaction with the terminating stage of a treatment relationship probably depends on the clarity of the goals identified early in the relationship.

To have a client return time and again when there is really no need, other than force of habit, could be viewed as overservicing. The health care worker may be taken to task by his or her peers—overservicing implies that the service is not being provided to meet a clear and reasonable objective. It may still be financially rewarding for the provider, but may not be providing any real or relevant service to the client. This dilemma highlights the importance of re-examining the good that is to be aimed for in any treatment relationship, which was discussed in Chapter 2.

If you, as a health care worker, are asked to do something you cannot or will not do, this may signal that your aims are incompatible with your client's aims, that the end (at least in part) of your treatment relationship is imminent, and that your client should be transferred to another practitioner. It may be useful to ensure that the client understands the full implications of what they seek, and why you feel you cannot be involved as their health care worker. When nothing more can be achieved by active treatment, the focus can properly shift to care and comfort. Health professionals find this particularly difficult when dealing with young patients,[52] but it can be difficult with many other patients as well. Team support in shifting the focus of care supports not only the patient but also the health carers.

Summary of key issues

- Mutual understanding
- Trust in the context of disclosure and care
- Privacy and social limits
- Risk and harm posed by carers or clients

Notes

1 T. Honderich (ed.), *The Oxford Companion to Philosophy*, Oxford University Press, Oxford, 1995, p. 380.

2 M. Spark, *Memento Mori*, Penguin, Middlesex, 1959, p. 140.

3 For a discussion of patient handbooks, see B. V. Corsino, 'Bioethics Committees and JCAHO Patients' Rights Standards: A Question of Balance', *The Journal of Clinical Ethics*, vol. 7, no. 2, 1996, pp. 177–81.

4 C. A. Berglund, K. Mitchell, and K. Cox, *Exploring Clinical Ethics, distance module in a masters of clinical education course on clinical ethics*, University of New South Wales, 2nd edn, pp. 195–6.

5 D. H. Flaherty, *Protecting Privacy in Surveillance Societies*, University of North Carolina Press, Chapel Hill, 1989, p. 9.

6 A. F. Westin, *Privacy and Freedom*, Atheneum, New York, 1970, pp. 6, 7.

7 Berglund C. A., 'Australian Standards for Privacy and Confidentiality of Health Records in Research: Implications of the Commonwealth Privacy Act', *Medical Journal of Australia*, vol. 152, 1990, pp. 664–9.

8 Medical Records Association of Australia, *Code of Ethics*, Medical Records Association of Australia, Canberra, undated.

9 C. A. Berglund, D. C. Pond, V. Traynor, D. Gietzelt, P. M. McNeill, M. F. Harris, and E. Comino, 'General Practice and Ethics: Listening and Understanding Concerns Raised by General Practitioners and Consumers', paper presented at the Fifth National Conference of the Australian Bioethics Association, Melbourne, 3–6 April, 1997.

10 Westin, p. 383; Flaherty, p. 5.

11 B. Andersen and E. Aranson, 'Iceland's database is ethically questionable', *British Medical Journal*, vol. 318, no. 7197, 1999, p. 1565.

12 Privacy Rule, Federal Regulations, vol. 67, no. 157, 14 August 2002, pp. 53181–273; such as C. Buppert, 'Complying with patient privacy requirements', *Nurse Practitioner*, vol. 27, no. 5, 2002, pp. 12–32.

13 National Commission for the Protection of Subjects of Biomedical and Behavioral Research, *Report and Recommendations: Institutional Review Boards*, Department of Health, Education, and Welfare publication no. (OS) 78–0008, United States Government Printing Office, 1978; and Appendix to Report and Recommendations: Institutional Review Boards, DHEW publication no. (OS) 78–0009, United States Government Printing Office, 1978, p. 309.

14 T. L. Beauchamp and J. F. Childress, *Principles of Biomedical Ethics*, 2nd edn, Oxford University Press, New York, 1983, p. 232.

15 Westin, p. 374.

16 Australian Law Reform Commission, 'Background Report No. 22', *Privacy*, Volume 1, AGPS, Canberra, 1983, p. 20.

17 B. J. A. Czecowoski, *Privacy and Confidentiality of Health Care Information*, American Hospital Association, Chicago, Illinois, 1984, pp. 1, 3.

18 Czecowoski, pp. 1, 3.

19 J. S. Mill, 'On Liberty', in *Three Essays*, Oxford University Press, London, 1975, pp. 92–3.

20 Australian Medical Association (AMA), *AMA Code of Ethics*, AMA, Canberra, 2003.

21   C. A. Berglund and P. M. McNeill, 'Guidelines for Research Practice in Australia: NHMRC Statement & Professional Codes', *Community Health Studies*, vol. 13, no. 2, 1989, p. 126.

22   *Privacy Act 1988 (Cwlth), Privacy Amendment (Private Sector) Act 2000 (Cwlth)*.

23   Principle 10, section 1(b); and Principle 11, section 1(c), *Privacy Act*.

24   NHMRC, *National Statement on Ethical Conduct in Research Involving Humans*, Canberra, 1999, *Privacy Act 1988 (Cwlth)*.

25   Section 95, 72(b), *Privacy Act 1988 (Cwlth)*; Australian Health Ethics Committee and Office of the Federal Privacy Commissioner, Review of guidelines under Section 95 of the *Privacy Act 1988*, Canberra, April 2003.

26   *PD v. Australian Red Cross*, New South Wales Supreme Court, unreported, December 1992.

27   World Health Organization, Alert, verification and public health management of SARS in the post-outbreak period, 14 August 2003. At <http://www.who.int/csr/sars>.

28   A. Surbone, 'Truth-Telling, Risk, and Hope', in A. Surbone and M. Zwitter, *Communication with the Cancer Patient: Information & Truth*, Annals of the New York Academy of Sciences, vol. 809, New York Academy of Sciences, 1997, pp. 72–9

29   T. Young, 'Teaching Medical Students to Lie', *Canadian Medical Association Journal*, vol. 156, no. 2, 1997, pp. 219–22.

30   *Breen v. Williams* (1996) 70 *ALJR* at 772.

31   'HIV doctor struck off', *The Daily Telegraph*, 26 August 1997, p. 5.

32   C. Shooner, 'The Ethics of Learning From Patients', *Canadian Medical Association Journal*, vol. 156, no. 4, 1997, pp. 535–8.

33   C. A. Berglund, 'Mandatory HIV Testing of Patients and Professionals: Bringing Ethics into Practice', *Medical Education*, vol. 29, 1995, pp. 360–3.

34   Centers for Disease Control, 'Revision of the CDC Surveillance Case Definition for Acquired Immunodeficiency Syndrome', *Morbidity and Mortality Weekly Report*, vol. 36 (supplement no. 1S), 1987, [inclusive page numbers]; P. Bacchetti and A. R. Moss, 'Incubation Period of AIDS in San Francisco', *Nature*, 338, 1989, pp. 251–3.

35   P. M. McNeill, J. D. Walters, and I. W. Webster, 'Ethical Issues in Australian Hospitals', *Medical Journal of Australia*, vol. 160, 1994, pp. 63–5.

36   G. Taerk, R. M. Gallop, W. J. Lancee, R. A. Coates, and M. Fanning, 'Recurrent Themes of Concern in Groups for Health Care Professionals', *AIDS Care*, vol. 5, no. 2, 1993, pp. 215–22.

37   J. W. Tegtmeier, 'Ethics and AIDS: A Summary of the Law and Critical Analysis of the Individual Physician's Ethical Duty to Treat', *American Journal of Law & Medicine*, vol. 16, no. 1–2, 1990, pp. 249–65.

38   S. D. Wall, E. W. Olcott, and J. L. Gerberding, 'AIDS Risk and Risk Reduction in the Radiology Department', *American Journal of Roentgenology*, vol. 157, no. 5, 1991, pp. 911–17.

39   B. de Vries and Y. E. Cossart, 'Needlestick Injury in Medical Students', *Medical Journal of Australia*, vol. 160, 1994, pp. 398–400.

40   Centers for Disease Control, 'Public Health Service Statement on Management of Occupational Exposure to Human Immunodeficiency Virus, Including Considerations Regarding Zidovudine Postexposure Use', *Morbidity and*

Mortality Weekly Report, vol. 39 (no. RR-1), 1990, [inclusive page numbers]; J. Jagger, E. H. Hunt, J. Brand-Elnaggar, and R. D. Pearson, 'Rates of Needlestick Injury Caused by Various Devices in a University Hospital', *New England Journal of Medicine*, vol. 319, no. 5, 1988, pp. 284–8.

41   R. Marcus, 'Surveillance of Health Care Workers Exposed to Blood From Patients Infected with Human Immunodeficiency Virus', *New England Journal of Medicine*, vol. 319, 1988, pp. 1118–23; S. E. Heard, 'Multidisciplinary Response of San Francisco General Hospital to the AIDS Epidemic', *American Journal of Hospital Pharmacy*, vol. 46, 1989, pp. S7–S10.

42   D. F. J. Mallon, W. Shearwood, S. A. Malla, M. A. H. French, and R. L. Dawkins, 'Exposure to Blood Borne Infections in Health Care Workers', *Medical Journal of Australia*, vol. 157, 1992, pp. 592–5.

43   K. Chant, D. Lowe, G. Rubin, W. Manning, R. O'Donoughue, D. Lyle, M. Levy, S. Morey, J. Kaldor, R. Garsia, R. Penny, D. Marriott, A. Cunningham, and G. D. Tracy, 'Patient-to-Patient Transmission of HIV in Private Surgical Consulting Rooms' (letter), *Medical Journal of Australia*, vol. 342, 1993, pp. 1548–9; J. Scott, 'Syringe May Have Held Virus: QC', *The Australian*, 30 August 1994, p. 3.

44   G. M. Dickinson, R. E. Morhart, N. G. Klimas, C. I. Bandea, J. M. Laracuente, and A. L. Bisno, 'Absence of HIV Transmission from an Infected Dentist to his Patients: An Epidemiologic and DNA Sequence Analysis', *JAMA*, vol. 269, no. 14, 1993, pp. 1802–6; A. Larriera, 'Doctors' HIV: Patients Will Ask', *Sydney Morning Herald*, 3 August 1994, p. 5.

45   J. Connell, 'Doctors Seek Powers to Test for HIV', *Sydney Morning Herald*, 5 April 1994, p. 3; A. J. Di Angelis, D. O. Born, and A. J. Hill, 'State Dental Boards and Mandatory HIV Testing', *Northwest Dentistry*, vol. 71, no. 5, 1992, pp. 33–5.

46   B. Lo, 'Clinical Ethics and HIV Illnesses', *Medical Care Review*, vol. 47, no. 1, 1990, pp. 15–32; Commonwealth Government of Australia, *National HIV/AIDS Strategy: A Policy Information Paper*, AGPS, Canberra, 1989.

47   S. Spencer, 'AIDS: Some Civil Liberty Implications', in P. Byrne, *Ethics and Law in Health Care and Research*, John Wiley & Sons, Chichester, 1990.

48   Mill, pp. 14–15.

49   J. Devereux, *Medical Law: Text, Cases and Materials*, Cavendish, Sydney, 1997, pp. 220–1.

50   J. Coverdale, 'Ethics in Forensic Psychiatry', in W. Brookbanks (ed.), *Psychiatry and the Law: Clinical and Legal Issues*, Brookers, Wellington, 1996, p. 67.

51   P. Burnard, *Counselling Skills for Health Professionals*, 2nd edn, Chapman & Hall, London, 1994, p. 103.

52   V. Sorlier, R. Forde, A. Lindseth, and A. Norberg, 'Male physicians' narratives about being in ethically difficult care situations in paediatrics', *Social Science & Medicine*, vol. 53, no. 5, 2001, pp. 657–67.

5

When the patient is young, old, or incapacitated

Overview

- Challenges to autonomy and consent
- Who decides best interests?
- Quality-of-life choices

The patient who is other than an adult, competent, participating client is discussed. For some health workers, these people are the bulk of their work. Particular dilemmas generated by the nature of temporary or permanent incapacity are canvassed. The role of the family in this situation is defined.

CHALLENGES TO AUTONOMY AND CONSENT

As a health care worker, you can probably sense when your clients have limited autonomy. They may seem slightly or grossly incapacitated (mentally, physically, or both). By virtue of their (temporary or permanent) incapacity, it may be difficult for you to ascertain with precision what they want, and therefore, to know what course they wish to pursue in their health care.

Sometimes there is no obvious incapacity. Rather, the client's limited understanding is just a product of the developmental stage of the client. Children are a large part of our population and a large part of health care work. They also present some of the more perplexing autonomy dilemmas for health care workers, as they negotiate treatment with both the child and their parent or guardian. Older people often lose a part of their cognitive abilities. If this happens, their care is similarly ethically challenging. Any of us can, at some point, due to injury, sudden debilitating illness, or emotional or physical shock, be temporarily or permanently limited in our autonomy. At such times, we also present health care workers with challenges as they go about the business of providing us with care.

In the face of these challenges, health care workers remain committed to the integrity of their clients. Sometimes, it seems as if these challenges prompt an even greater effort in this regard. Human rights documents express a commitment to upholding the dignity and wishes of individuals, regardless of their current capacity or stage of development.[1] How that dignity can be maximised, and appropriate care instituted, is the real dilemma of caring for people with developing or diminishing autonomy.

The discussion of consent and autonomy in this chapter is divided up into four areas: competence, information, comprehension, and voluntariness. It is designed to highlight how clients with limited capacity for understanding complicate the issue of consent and pose challenges to the health care worker's duty to uphold the autonomy of the client. This section should be read in conjunction with Chapter 3.

The formal components of consent, outlined in the following paragraph, are set by law. This is one illustration of the way law and ethics work together in setting acceptable standards. You will notice that the legal emphasis is on a minimum standard. On reflection you may find other higher standards. Law-reform processes, which are mentioned throughout this chapter, are a practical illustration of reflection on current standards, and debate about possible improvements.

The basic elements of consent are achieved when the client is

- competent (has the ability to understand what he or she is being asked to consent to)
- has the relevant information
- comprehends that information, and
- gives consent voluntarily.[2]

These elements are achieved best when someone has full autonomy, and is allowed to exercise that autonomy. You will remember from Chapter 3 that autonomy means self-rule. If people internalise this abstract concept of autonomy, they are able to set their own course in life and in health care, in a reasoned way that suits them best.

Competence: assessing the client's ability to understand

An assessment of the client's competence (their ability to understand the treatment on offer) is routinely made in health care, and particularly in aged care. A question about competence can be asked by nurses, medical practitioners, relatives, or other visitors. Each is monitoring whether the patient understands his or her situation and the options available. Despite the fact that assessment of competence is routinely carried out and is a vital skill, it has been the subject of few practical guides. One helpful list of issues to consider has been formulated by a team of clinicians and ethicists, which you can pose as questions to consider the circumstances of each patient:

- conducive environment and conducive frame of mind for decision making

- extent of cognitive function and stability over time
- adequate information available to the patient, that has been given and understood
- view of health professional
- additional factors relating to social situation and family.[3]

These questions clearly go beyond a simple 'mini-mental examination' of the patient, which focuses on the patient's orientation to time and place (and awareness of environment), to the environmental constraints on competence and decision making.

The rule of thumb is that it is rare for people to be incompetent for all decisions they must make. The competency of any particular client should be assessed in respect of their current circumstances and the specific decision that faces them—consent is consent to a specific treatment. This is recognised at law.[4]

This routine assessment of competence is ethically critical. Without competence, a person cannot give valid consent. If competence is limited, then there are limits to what a person can consent to. The limits generally are that only minimally risky and minimally invasive procedures can be consented to. That is because someone must be capable of making a decision before they can be judged to have made it. Under law, a capacity to understand a proposed procedure, when considered in conjunction with age and maturity, and by implication the capacity to make a reasoned decision given that understanding, may satisfy a requirement of competence.[5]

In the current ethical climate, the development of autonomy tends to be encouraged. For instance, children—particularly mature minors (usually children over 14 years)—can consent to minor procedures alone. In medical decisions there is a tendency to adopt a midpoint, at 12 or 14 years, below which children are assumed to be incompetent, unless proven otherwise. Above the midpoints, more responsibility of children for decisions is encouraged. These trends indicate the emergence of the view that children have a right to seek treatment autonomously.[6] The United Nations Convention on the Rights of the Child states that, given 'sufficient maturity', each child should be allowed to make autonomous choices on matters that concern him or her.[7] This notion that the right of the child to autonomy should be upheld is also part of common law, the law that is built up through judgments handed down by courts.

> The common law can, and should, keep pace with the times ... the legal right of a parent to the custody of a child ends at the eighteenth birthday: and even up to then, it is a dwindling right which the courts will hesitate to enforce against the wishes of the child, and the more so the older he is. It starts with the right of control and ends with little more than advice.[8]

We recognise that a child's autonomy over their own lives and body continually develops. It would, therefore, make ethical sense, as they grow older, gradually, to place increasing reliance on their expressed wishes.

This may mean relying on assent, or agreement, even if these would not otherwise be sufficient to meet the criteria of consent.

In relation to mature clients, it is also possible to place reliance on particular indications of assent or agreement. This is similar to a maximisation of competence in the case of children; it allows appropriate decisions to be made by the client, given capacity for reasoning and understanding of likely risks and benefits.

Exercise 5.1 Developing autonomy

There are ethical and legal grey areas in many aspects of children's maturity towards decision making. One quandary illustrates this. Imagine a minor who has not yet exercised decision-making capacity for herself, yet when, by virtue of becoming pregnant and having a child, finds herself assuming decision-making responsibilities for her child. In a paper written with legal academic John Devereux, we argue that developing and supporting the minor is a high priority, as the minor's competence is crucial to ethically rigorous decision processes for herself and her own child.[9]

As a tutorial exercise, map all the decisions you can think of that a child of about 13 years, who is in this situation, will be asked to make in the few months leading up to the birth, and the few months afterwards. Write a corresponding checklist of ethics concerns for each of those decisions.

Does the client have the relevant information?

Information is essential in the consent process. You should ask whether your client is able to access information, and then whether he or she is able to understand it. You may be able to assist in that process by presenting the information in a readily understandable fashion. The amount of information that clients are able to understand, the level of difficulty with which they can cope, and the effect of the way it is presented are all the subject of considerable research, even in relation to competent patients.[10] Of course, such issues become even more crucial when dealing with people of limited competence.

Some research on children's consent capabilities has shown that if information is presented in a personalised way, children understand it much more readily. Rag dolls can be used to demonstrate how blood would be taken, for instance.[11] Other techniques that do not assume that the client has developed abstract cognitive abilities could also be used, and to encourage them to elicit relevant information for themselves, children should be given ample opportunity to ask any questions they like.[12]

Health care teams constantly discuss how to resolve child and family best interests, particularly when there are conflicts with developing autonomy, lack of compliance with treatment regimes, and family rejection of treatment advice.[13] Developing capability for decision making can be viewed as complicating already complex treatment issues, but is a necessary ethics process.

The gravity of decisions makes a difference as to whether a mature minor is deemed capable of making a competent decision. For instance, in 1999, a 15-year-old active girl became ill suddenly, and required a heart transplant in order to survive. Her refusal of the transplant was overridden by a High Court judge, who deemed she was 'too overwhelmed' to make that informed decision. He approved the operation on grounds of best interests.

Exercise 5.2 Expressed wishes and capacity

As a group exercise, discuss what you would do when faced with her reported expressed wish: 'It's hard to take it all in. I feel selfish. If I had the transplant I wouldn't be happy. If I were to die my family would be sad. Death is final—I know I can't change my mind. I don't want to die, but I would rather die than have the transplant, and have someone else's heart, I would rather die with 15 years of my own heart'.[14]

Once the legal ruling was explained to her, M gave her consent. The presiding judge, Johnson J, said in judgment, 'M will live with the consequences of my decision, in a very striking sense…There is the risk too that she will carry with her for the rest of her life resentment about what has been done to her'.[15]

Is the consent voluntary?

Voluntariness is the final component of consent. People can feel coerced into agreeing, and this is particularly so for people with limited capacity, as they tend to be dependent on others. Children can feel unable to disagree with the suggestions of their parents or health care workers. Similarly, the aged and frail can have difficulty disagreeing with or questioning their practitioners or guardians.[16]

Establishing the extent of capacity and competence is very difficult. There is some help in tests such as the mini-mental examination, referred to above, which aim to assess rational consciousness and reasoning ability at any particular time. When people are rushed into hospital and some particular treatment needs to be given urgently, this test is sometimes used to see if that person is able to consent to the treatment. If they are found not to be competent at that time, a relative's permission may be sought or an appointed guardian may be contacted.

Paul Appelbaum and Thomas Grisso are eminent commentators on consent to medical treatment. They completed a recent study of the abilities of patients to consent to medical treatment in two hospitals in Massachusetts and Pittsburgh, USA. Their sample included people who were hospitalised with acute, life-threatening conditions. Appelbaum and Grisso found that, like other patients, the acutely ill patients were able to give informed consent. Their judgement of ability to consent was made on the basis of the following four abilities:

- ability to communicate a choice
- ability to understand relevant information
- ability to appreciate the nature of the situation and its likely consequences
- ability to manipulate information rationally.

They used specific psychometric instruments (techniques developed to test psychology and cognition) to measure these abilities.[17] Their point is that even serious illness may not make people totally incompetent to consent. Their view would be that the ability to consent should be preserved and enhanced, because of its fundamental importance in maintaining the integrity we derive from determining our own lives.

Even if it is established that the client has limited capacity or competency, it may still be possible for him/her to make certain decisions. Social workers and residential carers whose clients are developmentally disabled advocate maximal autonomy for the client. There is recognition that this is necessary not only because it is part of pursuing the ethics objective of autonomy, but also because their own life preferences support physical well-being and social integration.[18] This recognition means that in the fields of social work and residential care an awareness of the importance of autonomy and empowerment may accompany ethics or philosophy training.[19]

In the context of research, we protect people with limited capacity by not including them unless the research is particularly relevant to them, or people like them, and research on other groups cannot answer the question specific to children and young people.[20]

As discussed in Chapter 9, there is a distinction between research that is for the benefit of the person or persons participating in the research (patients/clients) and that which is more for the general benefit of furthering knowledge. If research is not therapeutic (i.e. if it is not for the benefit of those participating), people with diminished capacity are less likely to be included. This is particularly so in relation to the issue of children.[21]

Therapeutic research is much more ethically acceptable than non-therapeutic research. Although how therapeutic benefit is defined is itself a matter of debate.[22] As a general rule, the individual's position, and the likely outcome for that individual of whatever procedure is being contemplated, is the crucial consideration.[23]

There are equity issues for children's inclusion too, particularly if a social assessment of likely compliance with a trial treatment process is low given the parent's situation or lifestyle. For others, there is the burden of over-enrolment in serial trials if there is particularly good compliance with treatment protocols.[24]

If a procedure is non-therapeutic, then the risk or inconvenience that may be posed to participants is strictly limited, at least in Australia and the United Kingdom.[25] In the USA, there has been greater latitude. There, if there has been consultation with the public, if the research is of significant public importance, and if it is conducted with the consent of the families of participants, a relatively high level of risk and inconvenience to participants may be allowed.[26] The limits placed on the allowable risk to participants in non-therapeutic research highlights the way that responsibility is shouldered not only by society, but also by families in circumstances of limited capacity. The onus of deciding what treatment or procedures are justified is on health care workers and on substitute decision makers (those deciding on treatment plans on behalf of the patient).

Yet, in one instance of apparent non-therapeutic research which received international attention, the storage of organs or tissues of children who had died, without specific consent from relatives, raised tremendous ethics concerns. Though stored, they were not examined or used, nor had consent for their removal or storage been given. The inquiry into the practice at a UK hospital centred on a particular doctor, but in the course of the inquiry the practice was found to be more widespread than one site or one doctor. Stricter guidelines were recommended for the retention, and consent for examination of organs was recommended to be mandatory. Many commentaries were written on the process of grief, and rebereavement for families, on discovering there was more of their child to be buried. Public trust in the hospital system and veracity of treating doctors was also questioned.[27] Clearly consent, and the integrity of carrying out research processes that have been agreed to, underpin public trust in any process that is beyond the care for the individual.

Health care workers are constantly striving to improve health care and the treatments that they make available to patients. Sometimes, research that is innovative pushes the boundaries of current medical knowledge to their limits. When this research involves patients of limited capacity, there is unease among the community and the health professions. Community, and ethics, debate was obvious when, in 1985, a newborn baby received a chimpanzee heart, in an effort to keep her alive. She died shortly afterwards.[28] You are continually forced to examine what therapeutic benefit you hope to achieve and what the good is that you should, and can, aim for in the situation you are faced with. This is fundamental to our definition of health care, just as it is being fundamental to the business of providing care (see Chapter 2). The belief that some good must be achieved is essential if a health care worker is to offer potentially beneficial innovative treatment. This belief often translates into researchers championing the cause of the research, as is illustrated by a British researcher commenting on a ground-breaking living-donor transplant, performed on a 21-month-old child: 'We presented it to a large ethics committee and convinced them, although there was hostility at first'.[29]

What risks participants are facing is crucial to the assessment: Is someone about to die if not treated?; Is their condition worsening rapidly?; Do they face endemic risks? The latter was a consideration in early vaccine research in which children in institutions were participants. The infamous 1970s Willowbrook experiments, vaccine trials for hepatitis, were conducted on developmentally disabled children living under care in an institution called Willowbrook in the USA.[30] It was claimed that hepatitis was endemic, and that therefore, the children were likely to get it anyway. The side effects of the vaccine were therefore judged to be acceptable. This is a useful example for discussion of acceptable therapeutic boundaries. In my experience, the original research article, an account of a process that led to so much ethical and professional debate, fascinates health care students.

The Australian debate over vaccine research conducted in Australia in the 1950s and 60s is mentioned in Chapter 7. In that research, orphans were given various vaccines, which had been altered to make them less toxic. The hope was that the babies would be protected from epidemics that were sweeping Australia. The major subject of recent media reports over these trials is the possible exposure of babies to risk (not justified in the documentation surrounding the research at the time), and the issue of guardianship consent to such research.[31]

In the ordinary course of health care, we have a parental obligation to children and a mechanism of guardianship for others with diminished capacity. Our society recognises that a person with diminished autonomy may not be able to make all the necessary decisions. Yet we can try to maximise their ability to make these decisions, which is what many health care workers do.

In the health care professions, where autonomy of clients is a highly valued ethical principle, and where treatment decisions depend on rational and competent patients being partners in treatment plans, health care workers have additional protective obligations towards people with limited capacities.

Substitute decision makers may be used when the client's limited capacity to understand the nature of both the treatment and the illness at hand means that their autonomy cannot be upheld to a sufficient extent. While the client's family can help make decisions, it does not automatically become a substitute decision maker for the client. Even a close family member will differ from the client in many ways, and therefore cannot replicate the values and personal choices of the patient. The best that can be hoped for is that an informed decision based on the best interests and broad life-choices of the patient will be made on behalf of the patient.

There are limits on what these substitute decision makers can decide. For example, the responsibility that parents have to make decisions on behalf of their children is, in effect, taken away when the procedures at issue are regarded as non-therapeutic and too risky. For instance, parents are limited in their capacity to consent to female circumcision, and tattooing, on behalf of their children.[32] Their power to make decisions on behalf of their children is also limited if it has been shown that they have acted against the child's best interest in the past. Society effectively reserves the right to intervene to ensure that the best interests of each child are upheld.[33] The ability of parents to give proxy consent for their children is, in essence, a safeguard to protect the well-being of children, and as such, it may be limited if the child's best interests would not be served. Yet, there is a dichotomy emerging worldwide, with trends in research participation promoting greater involvement of children in decisions, and legal trends for children restricting choices, and mandating parental involvement in certain decisions, such as in the USA, for abortion decisions. Intervention is generally more frequent for mature minors in mental health, or personality disorders, or life-threatening conditions, but is not limited to these. Donna Dickenson argues that the agreement of the older child is needed for effective treatment participation, so forcing treatment is problematic in a practical sense as well as ethically.[34]

Guidelines and laws relating to substitute or assisted decisions are constantly evolving. For instance, the Queensland Law Reform Commission has reported on assisted and substitute decisions made in relation to people with decision-making disabilities.[35] The emphasis is on maximising autonomy by assisting in the making of decisions and by enhancing the client's comprehension. Once these steps have been followed, substituted decision making can occur, if this is what is required.

WHO DECIDES BEST INTERESTS?

The guardians and substitute decision makers grapple with the concept of what is in the best interests of the client, if the client cannot make that decision. The decision as to what is in the client's best interests is also informed by the professional opinion of the health care worker. The best interests of the client are, put simply, the primary interests of the client in maintaining and furthering his or her health and welfare.

On occasions, questions of best interests are decided by the courts. A 10-year-old child was able to decide to donate bone marrow to an aunt of his who had leukaemia after the Family Court ruled that this was in his best interests. The risks to him were judged to be minimal, and the psychological benefits to him were weighed against these risks.[36] (Similar reasoning allows people to supply regenerative tissue for transplants to relatives.) The Family Court in this case assumed the role of guardian, as it does when there is a conflict of opinion over the best interests of a child. The crucial factor in a guardian's appraisal of medical situations facing their charge is the value judgement involved in weighing the risks against the benefits.

QUALITY-OF-LIFE CHOICES

Some professions work more with quality-of-life dilemmas than others. For example, rehabilitation counsellors engage a client in constructive discussion and organise social, emotional, and physical management plans to maximise quality of life following an accident, illness, or physically demanding experience (such as drug addiction). What they are aiming for is to maximise the health and the life choices of their client. Quality of life is a value-laden term. It raises issues of what we should aim for for our patients—what we should allow or facilitate our clients to aim for. This is addressed in Chapter 3.

Quality of life is a key part of an ethics model proposed by Jonsen, Siegler, and Winslade. They stress that quality of life is not just a summation of medical indications and of what the future has in store for someone physically. They argue that the value that a person places on certain aspects of their well-being and life is part of their experience of quality of living.[37] It is intertwined with an individual's perception and life preferences. Trying to assess this for someone else is, therefore, inherently difficult, and possibly fatally ethically flawed. The perspective that is used in determining quality of life is crucial: is it that of the sufferer or the health planner? Some commentators are particularly concerned that the self-interest of health care workers may skew the quality-of-life measurements made in relation to their clients.[38]

Quality-of-life measurement, and quality-adjusted life years (QALY) are measures of life expectancy, adjusted for disability and pain. They reduce complex social, and well-being, factors to a single score. Increasingly, narrative is being suggested as a better way of understanding such complex qualitative concepts.[39] The narrative approach to ethics examines stories told by patients or professionals, or experiences recorded in published material, to understand what issues are prominent from those particular perspectives. When QALYs are used to point to the relative successes of some treatments (and so to justify funding certain health programs at the expense of others) this generates debates about ethics. The use of QALYs was one of the highly controversial aspects of the Oregon cost program, which was mentioned in Chapter 2. There is also a concern that formulas developed for determining increases in QALYs in relation to a particular condition, may lead to false expectation of real benefit for all sufferers of that condition.[40]

When the outlook for a client is poor, there may, at some point, be a debate as to whether treatment should continue. When children are involved, this debate can be particularly heart-wrenching. The pain and suffering inherent in the child's condition, as key features of quality of life, and in the proposed treatment, should be weighed against expected life-span. The extent of the potential benefit is ethically crucial in deciding whether to continue with aggressive treatment (treatment that involves, for example, painful invasive surgery or other procedures causing pain and disruption to a child's life). Benefits should be weighed against risks. Prolonging life for a short time may not be a benefit that justifies as much risk as would the benefit of providing a potential cure.[41]

Exercise 5.3 Diminishing competency

Now, as a review of the issues in the chapter, think about a case story about Lisa and Martin, two people with dementia, who live in an aged care home.[42] Lisa's husband has died, but Martin's wife is alive and visits him regularly. Lisa and Martin spend most of their time together, and appear to believe that they are married, even wanting to sleep together at night. They appear very happy, apart from when they are separated by staff to their own rooms. Lisa and Martin's children have been asked about their views, and they have asked for the two to be separated at night. The staff feel they have to protect Martin's wife, and try to make sure Lisa and Martin are not together when she arrives.

Think about what issues this situation raises for Lisa, Martin, their families, and staff.

Concentrate on: competence, choices permitted, and veracity.

Summary of key issues

- Consent capability
- Enhancing and preserving decision making
- Competence to appreciate alternatives
- Information and packaging
- Comprehension
- Expression of choice
- Voluntariness
- Risk and quality of life
- Best interests

Notes

1   United Nations, 'International Covenant on Civil and Political Rights', in M. J. Bossuyt, *Guide to the 'Travaux Preparatoires' of the International Covenant on Civil and Political Rights*, Martinus Nijhoff Publishers, Dordrecht, 1987.

2   Similar components are described by C. G. Weeramantry and D. F. Giantomasso, *Consent to the Medical Treatment of Minors and Intellectually Handicapped Persons*

Faculty of Law, Monash University, Melbourne, 1983, p. 82. The components were established in *US v. Karl Brandt Nuremberg Code*, in *Trials of War Criminals before the Nuremberg Military Tribunals under Control Council Law*, no. 10, vol 2, US Government Printing Office, Washington DC, 1949.

3   P. Finucane, C. Myser, and S. Ticehurst, '"Is She Fit to Sign Doctor?": Practical Ethical Issues in Assessing the Competence of Elderly Patients', *Medical Journal of Australia*, vol. 159, 1993, p. 402.

4   B. Bennett, *Law and Medicine*, Law Book Company Information Services, North Ryde, 1997, p. 22.

5   *Johnston v Wellesley Hospital* (1971), 17 DLR (3d) at 139.

6   For instance, Law Reform Commission of Western Australia, *Medical Treatment for Minors: Discussion Paper*, 1988, p. 43.

7   The United Nations Convention on the Rights of the Child, 1989, was adopted by the General Assembly of the United Nations on 20 November 1989. It was ratified by Australia in December 1990—see Department of Foreign Affairs and Trade, 'Major Step to Protect Rights of Children', *Australian Foreign Affairs and Trade*, vol. 61, no. 12, 1990, p. 893.

8   Lord Denning, in *Hewer v. Bryant* [1970] 2 QB 357 at 369.

9   C. Berglund and J. Devereux, 'Consent to medical treatment: children making medical decisions for others', *Australian Journal of Forensic Sciences*, vol. 32, 2000, pp. 25–6.

10 M. V. Williams, R. M. Parker, D. W. Baker, N. S. Parik, K. Pitkin, W. C. Coates, and J. R. Nurss, 'Inadequate Functional Literacy Among Patients at Two Public Hospitals', *JAMA*, vol. 274, no. 21, 1995, pp. 1677–82.

11 J. Berryman, 'Discussing the Ethics of Research on Young Children', in J. van Eys (ed.), *Research on Children: Medical Imperatives, Ethical Quandaries, and Legal Constraints*, University Park Press, Baltimore, 1978, p. 94.

12 R. H. Nicholson, *Medical Research with Children: Ethics, Law, and Practice*, Oxford University Press, Oxford, 1986, p. 144.

13 C. Harrison and R. M. Laxer, 'A bioethics program in pediatric rheumatology', *The Journal of Rheumatology*, vol. 27, no. 7, 2000, pp. 1780–2.

14 P. Foster, 'Girl, 15 forced to have new heart', *Sydney Morning Herald*, Saturday 17 July, 1999, p. 19.

15 *R v M*, Unreported, Royal Courts of Justice, Family Division, United Kingdom, 15 July 1999. Discussed in K. Forrester and D. Griffiths, *Essentials of law for health professionals*, Harcourt, Sydney, 2001.

16 T. Grisso and L. Vierling, 'Minors' Consent to Treatment: A Developmental Perspective', *Professional Psychology*, vol. 9, 1978, p. 423.

17 P. S. Appelbaum and T. Grisso, 'Capacities of Hospitalized, Medically Ill Patients to Consent to Treatment', *Psychosomatics*, vol. 38, no. 2, 1997, pp. 119–25.

18 J. S. Newton, W. R. Ard, R. H. Horner, and J. D. Toews, 'Focusing on Values and Lifestyle Outcomes in an Effort to Improve the Quality of Residential Services in Oregon', *Mental Retardation*, vol. 34, no. 1, 1996, pp. 1–12.

19 D. Henry, C. Keys, F. Balcazar, and D. Jopp, 'Attitudes of Community-Living Staff Members Towards Persons with Mental Retardation, Mental Illness, and Dual Diagnosis', *Mental Retardation*, vol. 34, no. 6, 1996, pp. 367–79.

20 NHMRC, *National Statement on Ethical Conduct in Research Involving Humans*, Canberra, 1999, 4.1, p. 25.

21 C. A. Berglund, 'Children in Medical Research: Australian Ethical Standards', *Child: Care, Health and Development*, vol. 21, no. 2, 1995, pp. 149–59.

22 P. Ramsey, 'The Enforcement of Morals: Non-therapeutic Research o:
    Children', *Hastings Center Report*, vol. 6, no. 4, 1976, pp. 21–30.
23 Re *Jane* (1988) 12 *FamLR* 662 at 690.
24 H. A. Taylor and N. E. Kass, 'Attending to local justice: lessons from pediatri
    HIV', *IRB: Ethics & human research*, vol. 24, no. 6, 2002, pp. 9–17.
25 NHMRC, *National Statement on Ethical Conduct in Research Involving Humans*
    Canberra, 1999, 4.1 NHMRC; Medical Research Council, 'The Ethica
    Conduct of Research on Children', *Bulletin of Medical Ethics*, vol. 96, 1992, p. 9
26 US Department of Health, Education and Welfare, *Federal Register*, vol. 43, nc
    9, 13 January 1978, para 4110–08.
27 For commentary and discussion of this issue, see: R. Coombes, "Paternalism' a
    the root of body parts nightmare', *Nursing Times*, vol. 97, no. 6, pp. 10–11; an(
    M. Redfern, J. W. Keeling, and E. Powell, *The Royal Liverpool Children's Inquir)
    Summary & Recommendations*, The Stationery Office, London, 30 January 2001
28 G. J. Annas, 'Baby Fae: The "Anything Goes" School of Human Experimenta
    tion', *The Hastings Center Report*, vol. 15, no. 1, 1985, p. 15.
29 G. McBride, 'Living Liver Donor', *British Medical Journal*, vol. 299, 1989, p. 1418
30 S. Krugman and J. P. Giles, 'Viral Hepatitis: New Light on Old Disease', *Journa
    of the American Medical Association*, vol. 212, no. 6, 1970, p. 1020.
31 J. Walker, K. Lyall, and R. Hawes, 'Wooldridge Backs Inquiry on Guinea-Pi;
    Babies', *The Australian*, 11 June 1997, pp. 1, 2; S. Dow, 'Trials and Terror: Medica
    Ethics Under the Microscope', *Sydney Morning Herald*, 14 June 1997, p. 35.
32 For instance, *Tattooing of Minors Act 1969* (United Kingdom) and *Femal
    Circumcision Act 1985* (United Kingdom), both discussed in G. Dworkin, 'Lav
    and Medical Experimentation of Embryos, Children and Others with Limitec
    Capacity', *Monash University Law Review*, vol. 13, 1987, p. 193.
33 For instance, regulation no. 502, *Children (Care and Protection) Act 1987* (NSW)
    and section 60(B) of the *Family Law Act 1975* (NSW).
34 D. L. Dickenson, 'Consent in children', pp. 209–13, at p. 209, in M. Parker anc
    D. Dickenson, *The Cambridge medical ethics workbook: case studies commentaries an(
    activities*, Cambridge University Press, Cambridge, 2001.
35 Queensland Law Reform Commission, *Assisted and Substituted Decisions
    Decision-Making By and for People with a Decision-Making Disability*, report no. 49
    vol. 1, Queensland Law Reform Commission, Brisbane, June 1996.
36 Re GWW and CMW Federal Law Court, unreported, 21 January 1997.
37 A. R. Jonsen, M. Siegler, and W. J. Winslade, *Clinical Ethics: A Practical Approac(
    to Ethical Decisions in Clinical Medicine*, 4th edn, McGraw-Hill, New York, 1998
    p. 151.
38 J. Richardson, 'The Importance of Perspective in the Measurement of Quality-
    Adjusted Life Years', *Medical Decision Making*, vol. 17, no. 1, 1997, pp. 33–41.
39 A. Edgar, 'A Discourse Approach to Quality of Life Measurement', in A. Surbon(
    and M. Zwitter (eds), 'Communication with the Cancer Patient: Informatio)
    and Truth', *Annals of the New York Academy of Sciences*, vol. 809, 1997, pp. 30–9.
40 D. G. Fryback and W. F. Lawrence, 'Dollars May Not Buy As Many QALYs A
    We Think: A Problem With Defining Quality-of-Life Adjustments', *Medica
    Decision Making*, vol. 17, no. 3, 1997, pp. 277–84.
41 S. Leiken, 'A Proposal Concerning Decisions to Forgo Life-Sustaining
    Treatment for Young People', *Journal of Pediatrics*, vol. 115, no. 1, 1989, p. 19.
42 Parker and Dickenson, p. 144.

6

At the beginning and end of life

Overview

- Personhood and beginnings
- Genetics issues
- Abortion
- Treatment in critical situations
- Suicide
- Euthanasia

This chapter discusses the more dramatic ethics issues. Classical philosophical choices and contemporary comment are canvassed. The dynamic nature of life and treatment is acknowledged. The dynamic nature of personal, professional, and societal views on issues relating to the beginning and end of life is explored.

PERSONHOOD AND BEGINNINGS

At what point do we give life moral and ethical significance? Human beings essentially start as clusters of cells, and before that, as separate, yet potentially significant, elements of human life (single cells). The moral and ethical significance of life has been debated since the beginning of early philosophical thought.

The thirteenth-century philosopher St Thomas Aquinas spent considerable time studying the Greek philosopher Aristotle, who had debated form and matter. Aquinas's position was that the human soul was integral to the person. He believed that the soul determined what made an individual a distinct human being, different from all others.[1]

Modern philosophers continue the tradition of that debate. There is debate among some over whether life itself is an absolute good (the view that life is itself an absolute good can encompass the notion that even the mere potential for life is significant), or whether there is a particular point in development at which time human life takes on a moral significance.[2] Other philosophers, more controversially, argue that the right to life depends on the desire for life.[3] That may mean that only beings who are conscious and self-conscious and desiring have a right not to be killed. Such philosophers even suggest that, depending on when this consciousness begins and whether memory is associated with it, all people, at least up to age four, are without a moral right to life, as are those who, by virtue of some degeneration, lose consciousness or their capacity to be desiring beings. Other philosophers have suggested that the indicators of the moral significance of life are brain development and an interest in human life.[4]

Solving this ethical problem is crucial in relation to processes that intervene in natural human reproduction. In vitro fertilisation (IVF) is one such process. It involves the external fertilisation of cells, and then implantation of the cells into the uterus. In order to refine this process, research was needed on human ova and sperm. The risk of damaging cells, and of 'wasting' cells is everpresent. The moral value of cells on their own, and of early embryos, needed to be debated. Mary Warnock, who chaired the British Government's Committee of Inquiry into Human Fertilisation and Embryology, has written a seminal article on this early debate, which occurred in the mid to late 80s, at the time when the United Kingdom was pioneering IVF.[5] The Warnock committee reached a compromise on the issue of when personhood, and therefore moral significance, can be said to come into being, settling on 14 days after fertilisation. You might have a different view of when to begin attaching moral significance to life.

Mary Warnock's book, *Making Babies*, is an excellent essay-style summary of the history of reproductive technology and the choices allowed within that technology. She argues that it is a privilege, rather than a right, to have access to so many opportunities as science now affords us in making babies.[6]

Even apart from the issue of the age of cells and potential reproductive material, heated debates occur about the rapid pace and ultimate worth of modern technological reproduction. Feminist ethics has emerged as a forceful tool of analysis in examining what society is offering women in terms of medically assisted reproduction.[7]

In the early days of IVF, ethics classes discussed issues such as the creation and storage of embryos, and their disposal. Rules to 'flush' unused embryos at the end of five years prompted questions about so many embryos having been created, and the position of the embryos as potential children if their potential parents changed their minds about their creation. For example, couples who planned to have a child then decide otherwise, or they may have failed to establish successful pregnancy and have given up, or they may have separated and now have different plans for the embryos. You may like to consider the following dilemma.

Exercise 6.1 Choices and limbo

In 1992, in the USA, a court case occurred to decide if a divorced woman could use embryos that she and her former husband had created and lodged with a clinic. Her former husband (the potential father) did not want this to happen. One newspaper headline at the time read 'Frozen Embryos in Legal Limbo'. The case prompted debate on rights to procreation, and rights to avoid procreation. The rights of the embryos to life were not established, as the embryos (a cluster of cells essentially) were classified as having a legal status somewhere between property and persons. The decision over whether or not they should develop to their full potential was thought to lie with the donors.[8] Similar cases have since appeared in other countries, some in circumstances of sperm and/or ovum being stored, prior to fertilisation. Does the fertilisation make a difference to your reaction to the significance of the stored cells?

IVF and related technology has certainly led to a myriad of ethics dilemmas, by virtue of the availability of viable and reproducible human cells. Embryonic stem cell research has captured the world's attention, as it involves complex and provocative ethics issues. Stem cells are cells which can develop into any type of cell. They are embryonic in coming from an embryo, but also in terms of their undifferentiated form. The technology now exists to harvest embryonic stem cells from embryos, then implant them into other tissues to research development of the cells into all manner of human cells. The proposal is that the cell regeneration could aid in management of diabetes, Alzheimer's, Parkinson's conditions, and possibly even with spinal cord injuries by generating fresh fully functioning cells for affected organs and tissues. The consequence of harvesting for the embryo would be that it did not survive. So, the debate has been about the intentional production of the embryonic material, and about the use of those created for another purpose. The concepts of personhood are central to the debate.

In the USA, there was extensive media coverage of the Presidential decision on stem cell research in late 2001, and ethics and religious advice on the issue. President Bush decided on a compromise: to allow federal funding for research on embryonic stem cell lines already created out of 'spare' embryos no longer planned to be used for IVF, but not to allow further stem cell lines to be created out of intentional production of embryos for that purpose.[9] It was a compromise that would not satisfy religious objectors to any use of human life for other ends, nor the scientists and researchers seeking full research flexibility. The Catholic Church always opposed IVF, as it increased the risk of disrespect for each individual life potentiality.

The UK is the only country that currently allows human embryos to be knowingly created for research purposes, including cloning technique and stem cell research by licensed researchers. It is permitted up to 14 days after fertilisation, as in IVF research, when the primitive streak appears.[10]

Other countries have had similar rigorous debates, and alternative cell methods, such as harvesting specified adult stem cells have been supported. These are differentiated, and specific in function to a specific type of tissue. It may also be possible, though more difficult, to culture cells from one part of the body and transplant them to other damaged sections, such as from a thigh muscle to a heart.[11] In a way, the ethics debates prompt alternative methods of therapy to be explored.

Exercise 6.2 Creation for others

The manipulation of life and of people's lives is at the heart of the personhood debate. The following example provides a useful opportunity for reflection on the creation of and respect for human life. A story reported in the world's media in 1991 captured attention and focused debate on what the limits are for a family trying to help their dying child. A *Time* magazine article recounted how a couple had conceived a child (Marissa) in the hope that she would provide compatible bone marrow for a transplant to save an elder sibling (Anissa) who was suffering from a form of leukaemia.[12] The ethics of conceiving a child for that purpose, and more generally, of using family members as live donors, were touched on in the media, and were debated actively by health care workers and ethicists.

The case of Marissa and Anissa Ayala is particularly challenging because it forces us to consider the sanctity of life. Marissa would not have been conceived if Anissa's life had not been threatened. Is it acceptable to use, or at least manipulate, life in that way? How important is the obligation to care for Marissa and Anissa? How far should Anissa's autonomy extend, and Marissa's, and the family's? As part of your reflection, make a list of the benefits and drawbacks of this bone-marrow transplant. Make separate lists for Marissa, Anissa, and their family, and the community.

BENEFITS
Marissa

....

....

....

Anissa

....

....

....

Family

....

....

....

Community

....

....

....

DRAWBACKS

Marissa

....

....

....

Anissa

....

....

....

Family

....

....

....

Community

....

....

....

Once you have your lists, try to decide whether the pluses outweigh the minuses. The crucial item on your list that makes you decide in favour or against the procedure is likely to shed light on what fundamental principles are important to you, and what ethical framework you prefer to use.

There is more on the theory of ethical frameworks in Chapter 10. Even before you read that chapter though, you could try to work out whether you are, for instance, more comfortable with deontological or utilitarian theories (see Chapter 3 for a discussion of these theories). You may remember, from Chapter 3, that the deontologist is an absolutist. The deontologist decides what fundamental obligation is the most important— such as right to life, or right to freedom—and whether a proposed action violates that rule or 'deon'. A utilitarian, on the other hand, weighs up the outcome of any action or situation, and then decides whether it is permissible, or what action should be undertaken. A utilitarian takes care to choose the action that is likely to yield the greatest good for the greatest number. The fundamental concern of each utilitarian is reflected in what he or she uses as a measure of 'good'—for example, happiness, or health.

Deciding issues of personhood is fundamental in both critical-situation dilemmas, and beginning-of-life quandaries. It is worth spending time on working out which of the philosophical stances you agree with. This will, in large part, determine your reaction to the dilemmas posed by the specific issues that follow in this chapter: genetics issues, abortion, treatment in critical situations, suicide, and euthanasia.

GENETICS ISSUES

An international genetic project has studied the genetic composition of the human race. Called the 'human genome project', its aim is to describe, or map, the human genetic structure, with an aim to determine what genes are responsible for what physical and behavioural characteristics. All human chromosomes carry DNA (deoxyribonucleic acid), and the human genome project is analysing and sequencing this DNA. An international group, the Human Genome Organisation, has coordinated funding and scientific efforts.[13] The long-term aim is to improve the health of all individuals, but minority groups are asking whether this project will result in benefits for them. Many others are asking whether it is dangerous to understand too well exactly what we are made of, as that brings with it the possibility that someone or some people will control other people or all humans.

As more about genes are understood, the issue of predictive genetic testing, availability of genetic information, and the possibility of discrimination or inequitable treatment in a social sense is vigorously debated. Genetic information is generally the subject of privacy protection, and inquiries are held into implications for employment, insurance (in which risk assessment is vital), law enforcement, and database management.[14]

Exercise 6.3 Genetic prediction

A simple genetic test kit was available in health related lifestyle shops in the UK. For about one hundred pounds, nine genetically determined metabolism processes for your body could be analysed. The focus was on diet and life-style. In the USA, a combined genetic based test of predisposition to osteo-porosis, heart disease, and immune deficiency is available through primary care practices. It is available worldwide through the internet.[15] Commercial genetic testing is the subject of guidelines, but these vary in different countries.[16]

In a small group, consider whether you would be happy to have these tests available at all, and if so, whether they should be available:

- in a shop setting
- in a practice setting
- via the internet.

List your reasons for support or objections in order from least to most strongly felt views.

Once an individual decides to have genetic testing, the information about risks they face or may carry in terms of genetically inheritable conditions, raises perplexing future decisions. Should they tell others or not, should they change lifestyle or further risk factors? The decision to have a test is generally accompanied by counselling because of the complexity of consequences that may follow.

David Suzuki has written extensively on the ethics of genetic manipulation of plant, animal, and human life. His 'genethic' principles are, in summary:

- to understand, in detail, the nature of genes
- to be cautious in claiming to understand the complicated interplay of genes in behaviour and 'defects'
- to accept variation as a natural and desirable phenomenon
- to maintain individual autonomy over genetic decisions that affect us as individuals
- to preserve the distinction between genetic species.[17]

The exercise below, devised as a tutorial exercise, can be worked through either in groups or alone. It is a fictitious scenario of genetic manipulation (and genetic testing) that asks you to consider the ethical importance of the genetic process, and to nominate who or what groups might have ethical concerns about the process.

Suzuki's 'genethic' principles can be used as a discussion base for the exercise. You could decide whether they should apply, and if so, what they would mean for the polis proposed in the exercise. Alternatively, other principles, such as those of Beauchamp and Childress (beneficence, non-maleficence, autonomy, and justice), could be used to examine the issues.[18] The ethical dimension of genetic manipulation is partly about control over individuals and species, and partly a scientific debate on what is most beneficial, in the long term, for the reproduction and survival of a species.

Exercise 6.4 Social genetic planning

It is the year 2100. A multi-national, multi-function polis has been established in space. Its job is to investigate the further use of space in light of the over-crowded and climatically undesirable nature of the earth. Advances in the human genome project (largely driven by Australian researchers, in particular) have enabled researchers to identify a gene that predisposes people to obesity. Obesity-related complaints would be undesirable in the multi-function polis in space, from which people will not be able to leave for the next ten years. Too many ill people will drain the resources of the polis to the extent that the project will have to be abandoned. The administrators propose either to limit work-permits to those who are cleared of the defective gene, or to rectify the genes of those with the obesity gene before they can gain work permits.

What do you advise should be done?

....
....
....
....

Is it a national or international problem?

....
....
....
....

Should the polis go ahead?

....
....
....
....

Should Suzuki's 'genethic' principles apply?

....
....
....
....

What would be allowed under your country's guidelines for gene therapy?

....

....

....

....

Using the following justice models, advise how a genetic testing service could be distributed: justice as fairness, comparative justice, and distributive justice. You may wish to come up with different advice for each model, or you may wish to combine the models in producing your advice.

....

....

....

....

....

....

....

This works well as an exercise in determining what is a good that the society, or international community, agrees with, and then how that good should be distributed. As your good, you can use either the genetic testing for the gene, or the genetic manipulation of defective genes. You may like to look back over Chapter 2, particularly the discussions of resources and justice, before you try this exercise.

Apart from examining, understanding, and 'rectifying' genes, we are also on the threshold of replication of entire genetic structures. This scientific advance, termed cloning, was reported in the media and captured the world's attention.[19] Since 1997, with the creation of Dolly, the sheep cloned from another sheep, the ethics of creation and recreation of exact copies of individual humans has been discussed and debated. Dolly was created 'by transferring the nucleus from an udder cell into an egg whose DNA had been removed'.[20] Many countries around the world were prompted to inquire into the process and the reason for it, and to ask what the ethical limits of such a process were. Should it be allowed at all, and should it be extended to humans? In the USA, President Clinton was very quick to promote public and government debate on the ethics of the process in relation to both animals and humans.

The US Senate Committee, formed to consider the issue of cloning, expressed a number of concerns about issues raised by cloning, such as the essence of personhood, the control over life, and the risk and harm resulting from the hundreds of failed attempts that preceded the successful creation of the perfect Dolly. They publicly stated that experimentation on humans would not be allowed.

The progress of Dolly has been closely followed, as has the progress and sudden health failures of other cloned animals. Dolly had premature arthritis in 2002, and progressive lung disease in 2003, which sadly led to her being put down.[21] Other cloned animals frequently suffer from heart failures, and generally rapidly ageing constitutions. Despite occasional sensational claims that humans have been cloned, the risk of creating many unviable and desperately malformed embryos and babies in the process, not to mention hidden uncertainties in resulting live babies, acts as a strong deterrent to human cloning.

Genetics institutes are working to minimise the impact that disabling conditions have on the lives of individuals. Further debate is needed on what should be thought of as a disability, and what is simply a part of the normal distribution and variation of characteristics in humans. The potential to develop a disability is also different to the actual development of disability. Should those with potential to develop conditions be thought of differently, and should they even be tested? Should such testing and information be limited to only what is socially and medically agreed to be serious and disabling?

Early diagnosis of potential genetic disease is itself an ethical issue. It involves assessment of family responsibility for genetic predispositions, and family ownership of genetic information, as well as individual autonomy and choice in investigating and controlling one's own health. Family members may well disagree among themselves on whether genetic disease is a collective problem or is the responsibility of the individual. The balance between the responsibility of the individual for his or her own health, and the responsibility of the family (or of society) for the health of larger social units, such as the family and society, may be different in different cultures. In a position statement on genetic testing, Kare Berg has outlined the importance of family responsibility in serious disease predisposition from a Norwegian perspective.[22] The balance between family and individual responsibility is not the same in all cultures. Nor is the broad societal availability of genetic information uncontroversial.

In China, the policy position that requires couples to follow their doctor's advice to limit children born with genetic aberration worries Western physicians and ethicists. The concern is partly in relation to the use of genetic information and reproductive technologies, and then applying it to concepts of normality and disability, and partly in limiting the parents' autonomy.[23]

The above exercise about obesity testing in a hypothetical work space-station of the future could be changed to include any number of potentially testable characteristics, in any work situation. Genes predispose us to variations in appearance (height, weight, hair colour, complexion, etc.), as well as to internal physical variations, not least in our internal organs (and their effective function), such as heart vessels and lung capacity.

The debates that occur constantly in relation to the ethics of genetics are a prime example of the often dizzying possibilities that science and health care (either singly or in partnership) present us with. The possibility of changing the very nature of the human race is increasingly real. Every now and then, the community calls for a halt to such developments, and asks for reflection on their ethics and legality. The overall aim is to prevent losing control of our future to technology. The community seeks to agree on particular objectives for technology so that technology can be harnessed, through agreed means, for those agreed aims. In setting these objectives and means we can take into account the concerns of both deontologists (in relation to the process of change) and consequentialists (in relation to acceptable outcomes).

ABORTION

The issues of sexual activity, planning children, and pregnancy face most adults, and they test our ethical convictions in our personal lives and our health care work. These issues may raise the dilemmas of preventing or aborting pregnancies for medical, emotional, or social reasons. The following scenario could be used to ponder the ethical choices raised by pregnancy.

Exercise 6.5 Personal choices and individual differences

A married couple has been trying, for some time, to have a child. The woman is in her early forties. At last, they conceive a child. The routine ultrasound at sixteen weeks reveals a very high chance of both Down's syndrome and various disabilities in the child. The couple pursue further tests, which confirm that the child is severely disabled. They now feel torn between their strong desire to have and raise this child, whatever its disabilities, and the fear that they may inflict a life of pain and burden on the child by allowing it to progress to term and be born.

You may wonder whether Down's syndrome should be thought of as a 'disability', and you may wish to know precisely what the other diminished capacities are. Some medically defined disabilities may not be considered disabilities in other contexts, and vice versa.

What would you do in the scenario?

The cultural context of such decisions may make a significant difference.

Abortion and contraception laws in each country reflect cultural stances and beliefs on the ethics of reproduction choices and the development of personhood. In some cultures, such as in China, abortion is officially seen as part of the range of contraception available. This is based on the belief that a human being or person comes into being at birth, not before. The Chinese debate over abortion is about the acceptability of late-term abortion rather than the acceptability of abortion itself.[24]

Health care workers who deal with such clients in scenarios similar to those above will also feel that their discretion is limited by different laws, depending on where they work. Beyond that, they will make their own ethical decisions about whether or not to be involved. As mentioned earlier, in Chapters 2 and 3, if there is a service that an individual health care worker feels unable to provide, he or she should at least refer to someone who can explore the decision with the client.

It is interesting to note that the legal stance of each country and each state on difficult issues such as abortion may change from time to time. Also, key players in each side of the debate may alter their views. The *Roe v. Wade* court case in the USA made history in the 1970s, as the case in which a right to legal abortion was argued for and was won. In an article published in 1996, the woman whose right to an abortion was at issue in that case, Norma McCorvey, discusses her changed views on abortion.[25] She is now vehemently 'pro-life' (anti-abortion), in contrast to her former 'pro-choice' stance, and since the case, she has campaigned outside abortion clinics to stop abortion. One of the things that has reportedly made a difference is that she has become a fundamentalist Christian. This is an example of one of the features of ethical reflection. Over time, and given our understanding, convictions, and experiences, we can change our minds.

Two prominent commentators in the abortion debate, who use the paradigms of classical philosophy, are John Finnis and Judith Jarvis Thomson.[26] Thomson asserts a woman's right to choose, arguing that the potential to develop into a human is not equal to a human, just as an acorn is not equal to an oak tree. Further, she claims that a woman should have the right to choose to allow or not to allow an imposition on her body. She makes an analogy between this choice and the choice that a Samaritan makes in helping another. Thomson uses the, now quite famous, analogy of a violinist to highlight how one body may be justly or unjustly imposed on another.

> You wake up in the morning and find yourself back to back in bed with an unconscious violinist. A famous unconscious violinist. He has been found to have a fatal kidney ailment, and the Society of Music Lovers has canvassed all the available medical records and found that you alone have the right blood type to help. They have therefore kidnapped you, and last night the violinist's circulatory system was plugged into yours, so that your kidneys can be used to extract poisons from his blood as well as your

own. The director of the hospital now tells you, 'Look, we're sorry the Society of Music Lovers did this to you—we would never have permitted it if we had known. But still, they did it, and the violinist now is plugged into you. To unplug you would be to kill him. But never mind, it's only for nine months. By then he will have recovered from his ailment, and can safely be unplugged from you.'[27]

Thomson's point is that the woman faces a difficult decision: to allow or not to allow another human being the use of her body. She argues that the woman has a moral right to choose what to do, on her own terms, and in her own way.

Finnis discounts this argument on a number of grounds, not the least being that the concept of rights is a popular concept that is widely used and misapplied. In Hohfeldian terms, a liberty or choice does not equal a claim right, which implies an obligation on another to act. (You may remember that Hohfeldian rights were mentioned in Chapter 2, as were the distinction between liberties, interests, claims, and rights.) Finnis questions Thomson's reliance on a woman's right (to anything), positing that a right does not exist until it has been proven to be a claim right. The notion of when personhood begins seems to be central to the debate between Thomson and Finnis; the earlier the point at which personhood is said to come into existence, the harder it is to discount that being's 'right' or 'claim' to life.

Throughout the parry between Finnis and Thomson, the different ethical frameworks of utilitarianism and deontology are apparent. In utilitarianism, serving the greater good may justify inflicting harm on others, depending on the circumstances and on the consequences for the mother, the potential child, and society. Under deontology, intending harm is of utmost ethical gravity, regardless of whether a good outcome may be achieved. Bad actions cannot justify good outcomes. These theories are discussed further in Chapter 10.

Exercise 6.6 Two interests and one impossible decision

As a review of this section, try this further exercise, in a group if possible.

There seem to be increasing reports of conjoined twins. Tragically, in many instances, vital organs are shared and parents face the impossible decision of watching both slowly deteriorate in health, or agreeing to operate to separate them, knowing that at least one may die as a result. The religious background of the parents, the willingness of doctors to intervene, and the capacity of legal systems to make best interests decisions varies between countries. See if you can think of a recent example of a conjoined twin birth, and research what happened. What were the views of those involved? What happened in the end, and what was the reasoning that contributed to the decision?

TREATMENT IN CRITICAL SITUATIONS

In critical situations, health care workers think and act fast. Reflecting on potential dilemmas prepares you for how you might react, and what your options are. Taking on responsibility for treatment was discussed in Chapter 3. Emergency or critical situations make a decision to care quite crucial. Any other help available and the seriousness of the patient's condition make a difference in deciding whether a health care worker should attend and assist. The levels of duty to care can be debated in legal terms as well as in ethical terms. The commitment to help others (the good Samaritan principle) applies in such situations, and this means that even a practitioner who helps out without proper equipment and resources will, generally, be protected from being judged on the basis of professional standards that would otherwise apply. There is some latitude allowed the health care worker because of the immediacy of the situation.[28]

Exercise 6.7 Critical decisions

Try resolving this dilemma. The essential elements of this vignette actually took place (but the story has been slightly altered).

A prisoner is booked in for a minor operation. On the day of the operation, the prisoner is transported from jail to the hospital in a prison van with two corrective services officers in attendance. The hospital is undergoing extensive renovations, and the parking close to the hospital is very tight. The prison van is parked a block away from the hospital, and the corrective services officers accompany the prisoner, soon to be patient, on foot to the hospital. At the corner of the hospital block, just after crossing a road, the prisoner attempts to escape. He runs away from the hospital, not back across the road, but down a side street. He is shot by one of the corrective services officers, and is taken to the hospital.

What should he be treated for?

....

....

....

....

Do you think his consent to the original operation is still valid?

....

....

....

....

Should he be treated for only the gunshot wound?

....

....

....

....

What should the health care workers do?

....

....

....

....

A choice must often be made about whether or not to resuscitate a patient. Some commentators lament the fact that cardiopulmonary resuscitation (CPR) is being increasingly used in all hospital deaths; so much so that people are not being allowed to die. Intervention could be seen to be prolonging suffering and doing harm in what often seem to be inevitable deaths. Laws are sometimes passed in some jurisdictions to excuse health care workers from the obligation to resuscitate patients who can be classified as Do Not Resuscitate (DNR).[29] In general, these reforms stipulate that, where a patient has rapidly diminishing lung or heart functions, care and comfort may be given instead of CPR (or other resuscitation techniques). This is ethically important. The imminent death of a patient does not excuse health care workers from offering help, but the goal of this help may not be saving life.

Advance directives are increasingly being sought from patients whose condition makes it likely that they will lapse into a critical situation. Their autonomy continues to be important, and what they would wish in particular clinical circumstances is taken into account. Just as is the case with consent, however, their expression of choice needs to be specific. Advance directives can be difficult to accept because, although a patient may express what he or she would like to happen given a particular situation, the unpredictability of symptoms means that the patient may not be able to grasp the true nature of what it would be like for them if that situation did come about. This means that the validity of carrying out their wishes when such a situation does arise is questionable.

When no specific directive has been given, clinical judgement, and the 'guardian process', may substitute. The best course is chosen in consultation with the health care workers working with that particular patient. The practice of patients providing advance directives relies on the assumption that a competent patient is able to choose whether or not to undergo further treatment, including life-sustaining treatment. 'Living wills' mandate which treatments patients do or do not want, and are prepared ahead of time to be used if the patient becomes 'incompetent'.[30]

Exercise 6.8 Tragedy and further choices

An interesting combination of ethics issues has been debated in various countries when married men die from sudden illness or traumatic injury, and their wives seek to obtain semen from them before they die, store the semen in an IVF facility, then use the semen to conceive a child at a later date. See if you can list what sorts of ethics issues the following scenario raises.

In 1995, Mary's husband became suddenly ill from meningitis and died aged 30 years. Mary said they planned to have children, and asked doctors to extract and store his semen, which they did. Later, Mary was denied permission in the UK to use the semen but subsequently won a High Court case to take the semen to Europe and use it there, in an agreeable IVF facility. There, she conceived a first child in 1998, and a second, four years later. The birth certificate did not initially list a father's name.[31]

Think about choices and how they are made and expressed, and the process of reproductive assistance involved.

SUICIDE

Suicide is the killing of oneself. Arguments about whether or not suicide is a legitimate action tend to centre on whether a person should interfere with their own life. Arguments against the legitimacy of suicide often rely on the 'God-given' sanctity of life; those supporting its legitimacy often rest on the principle that one's own life is a natural extension of autonomy.[32] Both sides seem to agree that suicide attempts by 'incompetent' people, who by definition are not acting autonomously, should be thwarted. Depressive symptoms, for instance, can often be seen in people who attempt suicide. Health care workers whose clients are manifesting suicidal tendencies often intervene to treat or refer the client for their depression, to ensure their safety and to help them to return to competent decision making.

Exercise 6.9 Final plans

You may like to ponder the following dilemma. It was written as part of a study about ethics in the setting of general practice. The vignettes in the study were constructed in response to the ethics concerns of general practitioners and consumers (these concerns were determined from a survey).[33]

A 52-year-old woman has breast cancer with bony secondaries (the spread of cancer to the bones). She is not currently in pain, and could, with treatment, have a good quality of life for two or more years. She tells her GP that she will not take the medication and that, after getting her affairs in order, she is going to kill herself. The GP discusses this with her, and suggests that she seeks counselling, but she refuses.

Some six months later she is found dead in bed, having overdosed on medication prescribed for a recent hip fracture.

Suicide is no longer illegal in Australia, but aiding suicide effectively is. Do you think the doctor did aid the suicide? Is the choice the woman's alone?

....

....

....

....

....

....

....

....

The debate on suicide is explored further in the next section on the subject of euthanasia. Physician–assisted suicide is seen as one type of active, voluntary euthanasia.

EUTHANASIA

Euthanasia literally means an 'easy death', or a 'good death'. It has been hotly debated, particularly in Australia in the context of the debate over the Northern Territory law giving people a right to a physician-assisted death (*Rights of the Terminally Ill Act 1995* (NT)). The passing of this Act was followed by lengthy development of protective guidelines, before a handful of people used it to gain medical assistance to die. Subsequently, a private member's Bill, known as the Andrews Bill, designed to overturn this legislation, was introduced into the Commonwealth Parliament. Eventually the *Euthanasia Laws Act 1997* (Cwlth) overturned the Northern Territory law in the Commonwealth parliament. This Act made euthanasia equivalent to murder or manslaughter. The initial Northern Territory Act and the process involved in both its inception and its eventual defeat involved people at all levels of the community in active debate about euthanasia.

Exercise 6.10 Principles in regulations

The process proposed in the Northern Territory Act is represented in the flowchart below.[34]

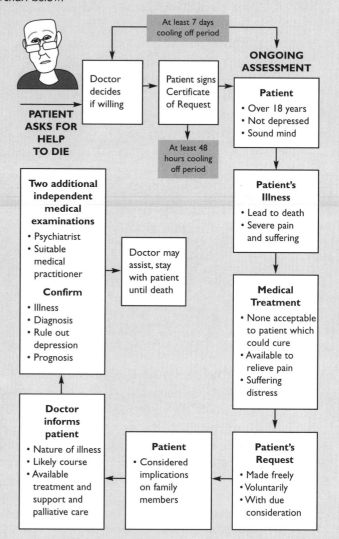

There is a sense, in the Act, of the importance of establishing that the illness of the patient is terminal, that it is the patient, and not some other party, who is seeking the 'treatment', and that there has been considered and slow reflection (on the part of both the doctor and the patient) in reaching what is, in effect, the final decision of a person's life. As an exercise in identifying the nature of the key ethical issues in the process (and the Northern Territory legislation's response to these), try tagging the boxes in the flowchart with the principles of beneficence, non-maleficence, autonomy, or justice. The competent and autonomous nature of the decision is a crucial link in each step.

As in any medical decision involving an ethical or moral element, the practitioner may decide not to participate in the process. As is the case in relation to abortion, if the practitioner does not wish to assist in the process, he or she would be obliged to refer the patient to someone who would be prepared to discuss or investigate the issue. This discretion is part of the notion of professional caring. It is up to each professional to decide what type of care they are prepared and willing to offer, in other words, to define beneficence in their own terms (this was discussed in some detail in Chapter 3). Beyond this initial decision on the part of the practitioner, the extent of the illness, and what can be done for the patient is a key consideration, as is the reasoned and informed nature of the decision-making process. Much of the debate over the Northern Territory legislation was about whether fewer patients would be asking to die if more could be done in palliative care to offer dying patients effective care and comfort. Even apart from the issue of the adequacy of palliative care, patient autonomy and patient perception of the extent and significance of their illness is a crucial consideration, whether as a safeguard that the decision to die is voluntary, or as the primary reason to allow physician-assisted suicide. These issues assume varying degrees of significance in the various euthanasia debates, depending on how much autonomy is valued in its own right.

Mr Dent was the first person to make use of the provisions under the Act, and his death was reported in the media. Although the first media report on his situation stated that he wished to remain anonymous, his name was revealed, and his explanatory letter referred to, in many subsequent media reports.[35] The general practitioner who cared for Mr Dent, Dr Nitschke, assumed significant notoriety, as he was willing to explain and promote the rationale of allowing an individual choice of this sort.[36]

Participants in the debate used key ethical terms in very different ways, as is demonstrated by a piece of research that is informed by a social constructivist perspective. By examining written comments and interviews about the issue in Australia, the authors of this article found that while key players in the Australian euthanasia debate relied on moral arguments, especially the concept of autonomy, they applied these arguments and concepts quite differently.[37] This analysis highlights the usefulness of reflection on the debate, as well as the importance of actually debating such a complex and emotive issue. Productive ethical reflection and debate does not only involve canvassing viewpoints: we also need to spend time defining terms and clarifying what we are discussing. Poor definition of terms is one criticism that has been made of the Andrews Bill. In particular, as noted by Cica, this Bill's failure to adequately define what is 'the form of intentional killing called euthanasia', may have skewed the debate.[38]

Euthanasia can mean many things; most notably, it can be 'active' or 'passive', 'voluntary' or 'involuntary'. Active, voluntary euthanasia, which is what the debate is currently about, is 'the deliberate hastening of death, on request by a person, to ease distress'.[39] In an early article on euthanasia, Anthony Flew argues that the will of even one individual who wants euthanasia can create a legal right to euthanasia. This argument relies on the importance of upholding a person's liberty, and on the suffering that would occur if their life were to continue.[40] Caution is often advised to safeguard against the possibility that euthanasia might occur in connection with less-than-extreme illnesses, or against the occurrence of active, involuntary euthanasia, in which people's lives may be ended against their will.[41] These concerns have been expressed in relation to euthanasia in the Netherlands, where euthanasia was illegal for some time, but prosecutions were not required by law. In practice, the regulations require patients to state their wish repeatedly and to have an ongoing relationship with their doctor. Then, the doctor seeks a second opinion, investigates alternative treatments, and seeks support from a committee of peers. The 'slippery-slope' argument—an argument that relies on the notion that allowing something in one situation opens the way for the same action to be used unacceptably in different situations—is often used in debates over euthanasia. Recent comparative research in the Netherlands suggests that there has not been an increase in requests for assistance over time.[42]

The form of euthanasia that seems to be implied by the Northern Territory Act, and that which was used by Mr Dent, can be called suicide. The procedure used by Mr Dent involved him initiating the process by pressing computer responses to confirm that he wished the fatal medication to begin to be administered. The doctor had of course aided the process by setting up the equipment and preparing the fatal compound. Physician-assisted suicide was precisely what Dr Jack Kevorkian, in the USA, wanted us to debate from the early 1990s. The first documented physician-assisted suicide that he was involved with was with Mrs Janet Adkins, an Alzheimer's patient who travelled across America to seek his help to die.

The article that first reported this suicide is useful for discussion.[43] The picture in the article shows the suicide 'device': three intravenous (IV) bottles connected up to a drip. The process is set up by the physician, then the drip is started by the patient pushing a button. The process begins with a harmless saline solution. This solution is then increasingly infused with two drugs to induce unconsciousness, and finally, heart-cessation and death. This article reports that 'Dr Kevorkian, a long-time advocate of euthanasia, said he took the action partly to force the medical establishment to consider his ideas. He said he knew he might face arrest'.

Exercise 6.11 Advice for professionals on assisting with final plans

Whether patients are entitled to ask for this help, and whether doctors, or other health care workers, should provide it, are crucial questions. Examining ethics-related codes can help you to identify the controversial points in the euthanasia debate. Take one professional code and one consumer code of rights and responsibilities, such as is set out in the Queensland *Health Rights Commission Act* (or in an Act of any other state) [44], and try to identify points of possible support or opposition to the action that Dr Kevorkian reportedly undertook. This exercise highlights the emphasis, in both consumer and professional codes, on patient autonomy. It also underlines the importance, in the context of euthanasia, of assessing how ill someone is, and whether treatment options are available or have been tried. The AMA's code of ethics states the following in relation to the dying patient: 'Remember the obligation to preserve life, but where death is deemed to be imminent and where curative or life-prolonging treatment appears to be futile, try to ensure that death occurs with dignity and comfort'.[45] There is a fine balance between allowing and promoting patient choices (and patient life-wishes) and bringing harm to patients. You will most likely discover that there are some principles which can be interpreted as being in favour of professional assistance in euthanasia, and others which can be interpreted as being strongly opposed.

Circumstances where the client is too young to express a choice, or is otherwise incapable of doing so, can generate debate that runs for decades. This happened in the case of Dr Arthur, which occurred in the early 1980s. A newborn infant with Down's syndrome received only nursing care and painkillers, under the medical instructions of Dr Arthur. Dr Arthur was acquitted of attempted murder, and a debate began over issues of personhood, disability, treatment decisions, and more broadly, euthanasia. The case is the basis of Raanon Gillon's book *Philosophical Medical Ethics*, which is one of the suggested further readings (see Chapter 10).[46]

It is perhaps not surprising that a debate over euthanasia polarises people's viewpoints according to preferred ethical frameworks. Neil Brown has suggested that the debate is characterised by a split between utilitarians, who may consider actions which, although concerning or even harmful, will result in a desired end, and deontologists, who will always act to preserve rules such as the integrity and sanctity of life.[47] More on these frameworks is included in Chapter 10.

Summary of key issues

- Personhood and potential for life
- Reproduction and medical intervention
- Genetic manipulation
- Community limits
- Abortion and autonomy
- Sudden, planned, or forseen end of life

Notes

1 D. Collinson, *Fifty Major Philosophers: A Reference Guide*, Routledge, New York, 1987, p. 34.

2 J. T. Noonan, 'An Almost Absolute Value in History', in J. Feinberg (ed.), *The Problem of Abortion*, Wadsworth, Belmont, 1973, pp. 10–17.

3 M. Tooley, 'Abortion and Infanticide', in J. Feinberg (ed.), *The Problem of Abortion*, Wadsworth, Belmont, 1973, pp. 51–91.

4 M. Lockwood, 'When Does a Life Begin', in M. Lockwood (ed.), *Moral Dilemmas in Modern Medicine*, Oxford University Press, London, 1985, pp. 9–31.

5 M. Warnock, 'Do Human Cells Have Rights?', *Bioethics*, vol. 1, no. 1, 1987, pp. 1–14.

6 M. Warnock, *Making babies: is there a right to have children?*, Oxford University Press, Oxford, 2002.

7 See, for instance, L. Le Moncheck, 'Philosophy, Gender Politics, and In Vitro Fertilization: A Feminist Ethics of Reproductive Healthcare', *Journal of Clinical Ethics*, vol. 7, no. 2, 1996, pp. 160–81.

8 'Frozen Embryos in Legal Limbo', *New York Times* article reprinted in *Sydney Morning Herald*, 3 June 1992, p. 15.

9 M. Hall, 'Bush OKs limited stem-cell funding', *USA Today*, Friday 10 August 2001, p. 1.

10 A. Plomer, 'Beyond the HFE Act 1990: The regulation of stem cell research in the UK', *Medical Law Review*, vol. 10, 2002, pp. 132–64, at p. 133.

11 J. Robotham, 'Thigh gives heart a leg-up and offers alternative to stem cells', *Sydney Morning Herald*, Thursday 9 May 2002, p. 3.

12 L. Morrow, 'When One Body Can Save Another', *Time*, 17 June 1991, pp. 46–50.

13 A. Campbell, M. Charlesworth, G. Gillett, and G. Jones, *Medical Ethics*, 2nd edn, Oxford University Press, Auckland, 1997, p. 73.

14 M. Otlowski, *Implications of genetic testing for Australian Insurance Law and Practice*, Occasional Paper No. 1, Centre for Law and Genetics, University of Tasmania Law School, University of Melbourne Faculty of Law, Hobart and Parkville, 2001.

15 D. Smith, 'Human genome project', *Sydney Morning Herald*, 27 February 2003, pp. 23–4.

16 M. Levitt, 'Let the consumer decide? The regulation of commercial genetic testing', *Journal of Medical Ethics*, vol. 27, no. 6, 2001, p. 398–404.

17 D. Suzuki and P. Knudtson, *Genethics: The Ethics of Engineering Life*, Allen & Unwin, Sydney, 1989, pp. 345–6.

18 T. L. Beauchamp and J. F. Childress, *Principles of Biomedical Ethics*, 4th edn, Oxford University Press, New York, 1994.

19 N. Hawkes and T. Rhodes, 'Human Clones Within Two Years', *Weekend Australian*, 8–9 March 1997, p. 15; 'Dolly's Cloners Say No To Families', *Australian*, Friday 27 June 1997, p. 7; H. Kuhse, 'Caution, Not Panic, On Cloning', *Australian*, 12 June 1997, p. 11.

20 E. Pennisi and N. Williams, 'Will Dolly Send in the Clones?', *Science*, vol. 275, 1997, p. 1415.

21 N. Hawkes, 'Arthritic Dolly is mutton dressed as lamb', *The Times*, Saturday January 5, 2002, p. 22; D. Smith, 'Cloning study points to early end for Dolly',

Sydney Morning Herald, Monday 11 February 2002, p. 6; L. Schlink, 'Dolly dies of lung disease', *Sunday Telegraph*, 16 February 2003, p. 40.

22   K. Berg, 'Ethical Aspects of Early Diagnosis of Genetic Diseases', *World Health*, vol. 5, 1996, pp. 20–1.

23   P. MacLeod and F. F. Clarke, 'Forget cloning and pay attention to China', *Canadian Medical Association Journal*, vol. 159, no. 2, 1998, pp. 153–5.

24   R.-Z. Qui, 'Bioethics in an Asian Context', *World Health*, vol. 5, 1996, p. 13.

25   *Roe v. Wade* (1973) 410 US 113; 'Abortion Hero Turns Pro-Life', *Sydney Morning Herald* [reprinted from the *New York Times*], 12 August 1995, p. 17.

26   J. Finnis, 'The Rights and Wrongs of Abortion', in M. Cohen et al. (eds), *The Rights and Wrongs of Abortion*, Princeton University Press, Princeton, 1974, pp. 85–113; J. J. Thomson, 'A Defense of Abortion', *Philosophy and Public Affairs*, vol. 1, no. 1, 1971, pp. 47–56.

27   Thomson, p. 48.

28   A. Dix, M. Errington, K. Nicholson, and R. Powe, *Law for the Medical Profession in Australia*, 2nd edn, Butterworth Heinemann, Port Melbourne, 1996, pp. 290, 310.

29   M. S. Lederberg, 'The Psychological Repercussions of New York State's Do-Not-Resuscitate Law', in A. Surbone and M. Zwitter, *Communication with the Cancer Patient: Information and Truth*, vol. 809, Annals of the New York Academy of Sciences, New York Academy of Sciences, New York, 1997, pp. 223–36.

30   J. Devereux, *Medical Law: Text, Cases and Materials*, Cavendish, Sydney, 1997, pp. 167, 168.

31   Based on article by L. Schlink, 'New baby from dead husband', *Sunday Telegraph*, 10 February 2002, p. 46.

32   T. Honderich (ed.), *The Oxford Companion to Philosophy*, Oxford University Press, New York, 1995, p. 859.

33   C. A. Berglund, C. D. Pond, M. F. Harris, P. M. McNeill, D. Gietzelt, E. Comino, V. Traynor, E. Meldrum, and C. Boland, 'The Formation of Professional and Consumer Solutions: Ethics in the General Practice Setting', *Health Care Analysis*, vol. 5, no. 2, 1997, pp. 164–7.

34   The key points in this flow chart are from 'Death with Dignity', sections 22–268, *CCH Australian Health and Medical Law Reporter*, CCH, Sydney, updated regularly.

35   The first media report was G. Alcorn, 'Mercy Death World First: Cancer Sufferer First to Die Under Northern Territory Euthanasia Law', *Sydney Morning Herald*, 26 September 1996, p. 1.

36   E. Slaytor and M. Lesjak, 'Euthanasia Seminar', *In the News* (newsletter of the New South Wales branch of the Public Health Association), vol. 11, no. 2, 1997, p. 7.

37   J. E. J. Oosterhof, J. L. H. Scholten Linde, R. Houtepen, and C. A. Berglund, 'The Interpretation of Morality: Cross-Purposes in the Australian Euthanasia Debate', unpublished Masters paper.

38   N. Cica, 'The Euthanasia Debate in Australia—Legal and Political Issues: Topics for Attention', *Australian Institute of Health Law & Ethics,* Issues Paper 2, February 1997, p. 3.

39   P. Baume, 'Voluntary Euthanasia and Law Reform', *Australian Quarterly*, vol. 68, no. 3, 1996, pp. 17–23.

40   A. Flew, 'The Principle of Euthanasia', in A. B. Downing (ed.), *Euthanasia and the Right to Death*, Nash Publishing, Los Angeles, 1970, pp. 30–48.

41 T. F. Murphy, 'Physician-Assisted Suicide and the Slippery Slope', *Department of Medical Education Bulletin*, vol. 3, no. 2, 1996, p. 1.

42 R. L. Marquet, A. Bartelds, G. J. Visser, P. Spreeuwenberg, and L. Peters, 'Twenty five years of requests for euthanasia and physician assisted suicide in Dutch general practice: trend analysis', *British Medical Journal*, vol. 327, no. 7408, 2003, pp. 201–2.

43 'Doctor Helped Woman Commit Suicide', *Sydney Morning Herald*, 7 June 1990, p. 12 (reprinted from the *New York Times*).

44 *Health Rights Commission Act 1991* (Qld).

45 Australian Medical Association (AMA), Principle 1.4(a) 1.6(a), *AMA Code of Ethics*, AMA, Canberra, 2003,

46 R. Gillon, *Philosophical Medical Ethics*, John Wiley & Sons, Chichester, United Kingdom, 1986.

47 N. Brown, 'The "harm" in Euthanasia', *Australian Quarterly*, vol. 68, no. 3, 1996, pp. 26–35.

7

Caring in an institutional and social context

Overview

- Community input
- Institutional limits
- Religion and health care

All care is influenced, in some way, by the institution and society in which it is made available. This chapter explores the opportunities for institutional and societal influence, and discusses the ways in which different philosophical standpoints identify different types of influences. Community consultation as a process of ethics debate is described. Guidance by moral or religious orders in the application of health care is used as a case study of the community and cultural influences on the ethics of health care. Particular choices made by professionals and clients in given institutional and societal positions are discussed in terms of ethics. The expectations of society are discussed and given prominence.

COMMUNITY INPUT

Community views are becoming essential to bioethics. It is no longer sufficient for professionals to define ethical problems, or ethical solutions, alone. Community views are being sought on particular ethical issues, and communities themselves are demanding to be heard on many ethics issues.

Communities are able to decide how much they support existing health care, progress in health care, and particular research methods. Their automatic support should not be assumed, as eminent ethics commentators, such as Hans Jonas, have been noting for some time.[1] In early and ancient history, there is poignant evidence of community input into professional standards. For instance, the Roman public rejected most experimental treatment on people who were seriously ill, and publicly castigated practitioners who undertook unacceptable experimental treatments, whether or not the experiments succeeded or failed.[2]

Many modern third-world cultures reject the notion of progress as it is understood in Western medicine.[3] Western communities may also strongly disagree with new medical technologies and treatments, on cultural or religious grounds. One example is the German community's opposition to human–embryo experimentation. The community objected to the extent that public discussion of human–embryo experimentation and related issues (such as euthanasia and organ transplantation) was stifled in the 1990s when philosopher Peter Singer visited. According to one commentator on the heated community protests that accompanied Singer's tour, the community's distrust of such research may stem from the Nazi abuse of civilians during World War Two, in eugenically motivated experiments on humans.[4] Eugenics is the altering of the characteristics of a population by a wide variety of methods. In this example the public reacted by stifling debate. The protests may well have been motivated by the hope that, without sufficient debate, human–embryo research would not go ahead.

While public reactions involving attempts to stifle debate may not represent effective community debate on the issues, the wishes of the community should nevertheless be seriously considered by researchers if a social definition of justice is to be accepted. Under a social definition of justice, community advice must be sought so that the benefits and burdens (of specific advances in health care) to individuals and the community are acceptable. As Douglas states, '[t]he public reception of any policy for risks will depend on standardized public ideas about justice'.[5] Frankel similarly considers that limits to professional choices, particularly in research, should be provided by social policy so that individuals are better protected from harms that are regarded as unacceptable by society.[6]

Exercise 7.1 New frontiers and personal views

Try this exercise to think about what you, and those working with you, would accept. If you are facilitating the group discussion, expect to hear different views, and encourage people to express those different views.

Transplantation of hands is a new procedure in this century, demonstrating how complex procedures are now undertaken with advances in transplantation medicine, and in precision of surgical technology. There are implicit cultural tolerances of body parts beyond organs being 'harvested' and used for others. Our tolerance of external body features is even being tested with mooted facial transplantation for people who have had devastating facial disfigurement. Compliance with anti-rejection medication regimes after surgery is receiving as much attention as the clinical complexity of the procedures, as the post-care process is long term and intensive as well.[7]

As a group, try to describe differences in what each of you would accept in different types of organ, tissue, and body part transplantation.

....

....

....

....

....

....

Identify cultural, religious, and personal limits to what each person would accept.

....

....

....

....

....

....

....

These discussions of different views are crucial in gauging community acceptance or opposition to new medical advances.

In the context of health research, little was known, until recently, about community views on, or expectations of, research.[8] There was a sense that research ought not to be pushed too far as it might disquiet the community, and there was a general consensus that there was a limit to how ethically risky research could be before the community would find it unethical. In a community consultation survey, respondents were generally supportive of research, but they were more conservative in hypothetically offering their own participation or that of children. Children were rather more reticent than adults in supporting their own inclusion in research that involved being subjected to more than non-invasive examinations. In relation to adults, the key finding of the survey was that the respondents could draw a line of acceptability and distinguish some research as unacceptable to them. In a way, this gives research above their line of acceptability a community mandate, and research below their line of acceptability, a community caution or even injunction.[9]

Chalmers and Silverman favour 'public consideration' of formal and informal medical research as a type of risk assessment, not so much as a community judgement of acceptable risk, but more because they believe that the community should take responsibility for the reality that progress involves some risk. They caution against the idealistic double-standard of wanting the benefits of research without the inevitable risk of harm that accompanies research. They would prefer the community to acknowledge that acceptable means for the ends of research must include risk.[10]

The Sydney survey discussed above supported two key safeguards that appeared to have the backing of the community. The first was the opportunity for community consideration of acceptable benefits and burdens in research. The second was informed consent on the part of each research participant. The safeguard of community input is partially fulfilled by the inclusion of lay members in ethics committees.[11] In New Zealand, these members must represent a community group, and be nominated and endorsed by the community, in the true sense of representation. The involvement of Maori representatives ensures that Maori values and perspectives are incorporated in research decisions.[12] Community consultation may be more obvious when medicine is pushing its own bounds— for example, in the recent public debate on euthanasia (euthanasia is discussed in Chapter 6). It may, however, be just as ethically important to seek community comment on routine aspects of health care, as it is to consult in relation to more dramatic areas, such as cutting-edge research and challenging areas of practice.

Even in routine health care, you may not be able to assume that you, as health care workers, know the type of health care, or manner of delivery of that care, that is appropriate for particular communities. In some cultures, such as South-East Asian cultures, there are strong beliefs about hot and cold water, and running and still water, particularly in the context of women in labour and immediately post-partum. These beliefs are very different to Western notions, and so we might expect very different attitudes to the use of labour-floor facilities. One research project on the attitudes of midwives to their patients found that the midwives surveyed thought that some Asian women were '"bad patients" who lacked compliance; made a fuss about nothing; and did not have normal maternal instincts'. The judgement made by these midwives about the patients was probably due to a lack of cultural understanding. Anthropological research is now bringing a greater understanding of cultural differences in the context of health care.[13]

Feminist research is similar in that it focuses on aspects of culture and power that define expectations and possible ethical behaviours, in the contexts of the doctor–nurse relationship, or the health professional–client relationship. Culturally informed research may well be a useful model for other professionals too. Until we communicate and listen to community voices, we won't know if our current system of health and health care practices is acceptable. In the case study mentioned above, until the Asian women were listened to, acceptable cleansing facilities were simply not available to them.

The community voice is not present in the jargon of either health care workers or ethicists, but it can be heard, if you listen. Hearing community views is important in, or at least is compatible with, many of the key ethical theories. In liberalism, in which there is little role for cohesive community control over individual actions, there is nevertheless a sense of a general community consensus on limits to autonomy. Libertarianism also implicitly assumes that there is some kind of community agreement and that there are obligations to endure certain burdens for the good of the society to which we belong. Within the framework of libertarianism, only a majority community view, the general will, would be the acceptable basis of a limit on liberty.[14]

A strong sense of community limits, self-defined by the community, is essential to communitarianism, a form of ethics that is gaining popularity in Europe.[15] In deontological theory, there is, at the very least, a minimum ethical standard that one would expect to be shared among members of the community, below which these community members would not go. In Kant's work, there is a sense that we should respect others, and that there should be a limit to how much we interfere or harm them, so that each person can develop his or her own moral self.[16] The concept of consultation is also compatible with specified principlism, which holds that principles can be identified, but that their meaning and application should be defined with reference to cultural norms or standards.[17]

Whichever your preferred ethical theory, and you can read more about the theories in Chapter 10, it would quite obviously enlighten you as health care workers to know what the community you serve regards as acceptable; to know, in other words, how much a client could ask for, and how much others could offer them or ask them to undertake, and still be regarded, by the community, as an ethical citizen. Further, if you regard the process of defining acceptable practices as a joint responsibility of professionals and the community, there needs to be a means of expressing views from the community, and you need to hear those views and communicate your stance to the community.

Exercise 7.2 Client and community views on practices

Try this exercise. Think about how you might hear your client's views on a vexing issue, something which seems to be at the heart of your health practice. Pick an everyday instance, such as queues to see you, waiting lists, or what you usually do first in a consultation. How could you find out the client's view?

The problem I am thinking about is:

....

....

....

....

I could try to find out the community view by:

....

....

....

....

....

....

In some communities, even asking for someone's name has ethical significance. In the context of drug using communities, health professionals sometimes forgo 'real' names so that their service can be received by people who would otherwise be fearful of attending a health care service. It is reportedly quite common to see 'Mickey Mouse' or other fictitious names on records. This only became possible when that particular community's fear of the use and recording of real names was acknowledged.

There are now legislative requirements for guideline-forming bodies within the ambit of the National Health and Medical Research Council (NHMRC) to consult with the community before formulating ethics guidelines.[18] The Consumers' Health Forum of Australia (CHF), which has gained recognition as the peak consumer body for health issues, holds places on many key committees that develop standards for health practices and/or research practices. Human research ethics committees (HRECs), formerly called IECs, which consider the ethics of research at the institutional level, have long had a requirement, laid down by the NHMRC, for two laypeople to be on each committee. Those people are assumed to be a link to the community. They, along with the other non-clinical members of the committee (a lawyer and a minister of religion), try to comment on research from the perspectives of the research participants and the community.

In processes of law reform, it is now common to undertake large-scale community consultation. There is frequently a public advertisement calling for submissions, and also active recruitment of people through surveys to hear their views on certain reforms that are being considered. In early stages of research in specific communities, such as the Aboriginal communities, it is common for wide consultation to be undertaken, as the research process itself is a collaboration, and must be in tune with cultural and community expectations.[19] Government policy making is also increasingly incorporating community participation in different sectors.[20] Have a look at the composition of the governing board of the health care institution you work for. You will no doubt find that there are some community representatives there. They have a say in setting the operating objectives of health care, and in defining the priority of objectives (prioritising objectives is addressed in Chapter 2). They play an important part in the scrutiny of the extent to which institutions succeed in meeting their stated objectives.

Given the value placed on community expressions of its point of view, there is caution when a representative view is heard. This caution has been expressed repeatedly in relation to contentious issues. For example, in 1990 community views on AIDS research were formalised by the AIDS Clinical Trials Group (ACTG) in the USA (the decisions made by ACTG have effect nationwide).[21] These viewpoints, called 'ACTG community positions', were subject to particular scrutiny, given the power that AIDS activists have to influence the availability and accessibility of treatments.[22] People began questioning whether the views of the gay (predominantly) white male members of AIDS activist groups also spoke for other sections of the community. So, the process of consultation is itself also the subject of ethical scrutiny.

Throughout this book, there is a theme of encouraging communication between professionals and the community on preferred ethical standards for the practice of health care, and this theme is explored further in Chapter 9, in the context of health care research. An opportunity for such consultation exists through the mass media.

The popular press is increasingly reporting on health issues, treatment, policy, and research.[23] It is a source of health information for the general public, and provides an opportunity for the community to comment on existing or proposed health practices or research. Media reporting on health issues can be seen as communicative interaction between, on the one hand, interested and accessible community members and professionals, and on the other hand, other political actors.[24] Its job is to reflect the state of society by reporting on current issues, which obviously include community concerns over health treatment and health research.

Indeed, there is such potential for the press to be successfully used by professionals in sending out particular health information that the NHMRC has issued the following warning: 'The job of journalism is not public relations for the health messages of the day. It is to question and probe and analyse'.[25] The danger is that the more successful the health or scientific community is in using the media, the less open the media may be to contrary views, or the less able it may be, by virtue of limited space to report other key community insights.

There does seem to be potential for the media, health policy makers, health professionals, and the public to become involved in health issues as they are presented for further discussion in the media.[26] However, this discussion is not necessarily explicitly ethical.[27]

Some inquiries can be prompted by media reports, such as on the immunisation trials on Australian orphans in the 1950s and 60s—these trials featured in the media a few years ago. The issue of the use of wards of the state for the research was of particular concern to both the public and to the orphans (who were unaware that they had been part of the research).[28]

In that instance, concern over the particular issue was expressed, and the issue was opened up for debate. It was then reflected on over time. Professionals, researchers, the patients, and the community were all involved in the debate. The process of reflection can often be traced in later media reports.

Current newspaper clippings can be very useful as triggers in learning about ethics. They raise interest in the ethics of current issues. Students often feel they know something about the issues, and can talk about them, and they often raise the issue of who should comment on ethics. This can lead to role-playing of which sectors of the community might have which particular concerns. Newspaper articles frequently concentrate on individual cases, and can thus be used as a vignette in class settings, allowing the class to consider a particular health problem and its associated dilemmas.[29]

The community view in an ethics debate is usually termed 'community input' or 'community consultation' because it is not seen as mandating professional behaviour. Community views could, however, guide professional behaviour by informing you of what would and would not be acceptable to any given client; given two morally similar (to you) choices, you might choose the path that is culturally sensitive and ethically preferable in the eyes of the community you serve.

Seeking community input is part of the dynamic nature of ethics. Standards, and the situations to which we apply them, can change. Re-examination of ethics issues, at times in partnership with the key parties affected, is likely to be an enduring theme of modern health care ethics. Community concerns highlight how we work and live in a society that is complex. We need to communicate with each other so that our standards are appropriate. We need to use the benefits that stem from pooling our ideas and resources, and as we each seek to use what we need from the societal pool, we need to be careful not to infringe on the dignity and self-respect of individual members of society.

Exercise 7.3 Decisions in community contexts

The following case focuses on the community contexts, and how inclusion in a particular community is a social and political decision. This case was drawn from reports of a deportation hearing in the UK.[30]

A woman from an African country travelled to Ireland. Once there, she applied for residency, on the grounds of political persecution if she returned home. Her application and appeal were not successful. During the course of the appeal process, she became pregnant. The woman then applied on behalf of her unborn child for residency for the child, on the grounds that the child would be persecuted in her home country. The deportation of the woman was delayed, and an expedited hearing was held.

Make notes on the issues you think are important in this case, what should happen in relation to residency, medical care for the woman and the child, and your reasoning.

....

....

....

....

....

....

....

The cultural and community context of treatment and ethics decisions is highlighted in a training program with the acronym C.A.R.E. for systematic personal ethics consideration for trainee physicians. C is for the physician's core beliefs, A is for action in similar situations in the past, R is for reasoned opinions of others, and E is for experience of others in similar situations in the past. Each item is critiqued as part of the ethics reflection, so the model is a shorthand to prompt reflection on reasonable options.[31] Notice that the model explicitly acknowledges the personal beliefs of the carer as well as the community context care is applied in.

INSTITUTIONAL LIMITS

Institutional goals and service expectations are discussed in Chapters 1 and 2, and will not be repeated here. Some specific professional responsibilities and limits, whatever the institutional context, are also covered in Chapter 8. Every institution has its own culture that continually shapes the professional work done within the ambit of that institution. The culture of peers also moulds ethical aspirations and standards.

Quality-assurance processes, and peer review, set up opportunities for institutions to refine their written protocols for service delivery and for the limits within which professionals work. Increasingly, institutions are encouraging staff to report positive events as well as adverse events. In terms of ethics, what works and what doesn't work in a system are just as important as how good or bad the people working within that system are. There is continual institutional reflection on safe and ethical limits within which members operate.

In addition, institutions operate under a state or Commonwealth umbrella. Comprehensive operating guidelines and expectations are provided by government health departments. Some examples of guidelines and limits in relation to the prioritisation of patients for admission into public hospitals are discussed in Chapter 2. Chapter 3 includes a discussion of safeguards in relation to medical records.

Operating guidelines have ethical assumptions built into them. These assumptions relate to:

- appropriate levels of training and skill for particular jobs
- what care to offer and how to deliver it
- social expectations of what would be a priority in particular situations
- availability of care.

Ultimately, an institution has to decide if it is meeting a need sufficiently, and if its employees are playing a proper part. If the work of an employee is falling short of existing standards, an institution may prefer to dismiss that employee, rather than allowing him or her to risk either the work of the institution, or the public's trust that the institution will provide adequate care.

RELIGION AND HEALTH CARE

Early Western writings on ethics were more obviously intertwined with religious philosophy and theology than is the case today. These writings struggled with the power of God, and the nature of man as related to the world and to God. Western philosophers transformed and challenged the Church, particularly throughout the Reformation. Doctrines about man's manipulation of life emerged.[32]

The religious philosophies of non-Western cultures are receiving attention in the context of health care ethics. Robert Veatch has written extensively on this matter.[33] Given the multicultural nature of many modern Western societies, it is increasingly common to find summaries of the implications that different non-Western philosophies have for health included in health (or health-related) texts. Some non-Western philosophies and religions give specific guidance on how medical practitioners should treat their patients. For instance, under Chinese medical ethics, which have Confucian, Buddhist, and Taoist affiliations, modesty and hard work are valued. Under the teachings of Islam, a practitioner should treat the person's body and mind, should encourage what is good, and should restrain people from doing what is bad. Virtue and equal treatment of rich and poor is emphasised, and certain rules are laid down, such as not procuring abortion.[34]

If you are religious, your religion can, and probably does, affect your work as a health care worker. It is one of the things that forms your values and how you try to relate to others. It would be artificial to try to have two moral or ethical standards—one religious standard for purely religious life, and one professional standard for professional work. In Chapter 1, religion was noted as one of the influences that goes towards defining you as an individual.

There are times when a religion we may adhere to prompts us to examine our place in current health practices, either as providers or as consumers of services. Abortion, euthanasia, and blood transfusion, are perhaps the most often cited examples (abortion and euthanasia are discussed in Chapter 6).

Commenting on euthanasia from a Singaporean perspective, Kamaljit Singh and Goh Lee Gan state that the vast majority of the Singaporean population is religious. The population, therefore, would react on religious grounds to euthanasia, or any other issue. These authors summarise the key religious views held by Singaporeans, as follows:

- Christians and Buddhists tend to affirmatively value both life and non-interference with life (Christians, because they believe life has divine origin; Buddhists, because they believe life has spiritual destiny).
- Muslims tend to view suffering as a mitigation of suffering in the hereafter, in accordance with Islamic law.
- Jews tend to hold the sanctity of life to be infinite, in accordance with Jewish laws.[35]

Any practices that challenge religious convictions can raise dilemmas for those holding those particular convictions. Any parts of practices that challenge religious convictions are also ethically suspect for those who adhere to those faiths. For instance, Jehovah's Witnesses believe that it is wrong to place foreign blood matter into a person's body. Thus, for strict Jehovah's Witnesses, any part in a process that aims to place blood or blood-derived products into people poses a dilemma. Therefore, problematic medical practices include not only blood transfusion, but any collection or use of blood products.

Exercise 7.4 Religious conviction and actions

Consider the following example, which was discussed in the Australian mass media in 1990.

A taxi driver was allegedly called to pick up a package from the Red Cross and deliver it to a hospital. The package contained blood. The blood was urgently needed for an operation, but it never arrived. The blood was allegedly found abandoned near the driver's taxi depot, packets pierced and unusable.

What do you think?

....

....

....

....

....

....

....

If the driver did in fact dump the blood, and tamper with it, did he have a right to act on what seems to have been his religious convictions that use of blood was fundamentally wrong?

....

....

....

....

....

....

....

Conversely, did those who gave it to him have an obligation to ensure that he was agreeable to delivering the blood before they entrusted it to him?

....

....

....

....

....

....

....

This perplexing hypothetical works well as a group exercise. It stimulates discussion of what the bounds of acceptable behaviour are, who determines these bounds, and whether it is community expectations or moral and religious conviction that should prevail. Bear in mind the fact that the taxi driver is not a health professional. He has not sworn to abide by a code of ethics. He has not agreed with the charter of the hospital. Yet he, like many other non-health professionals, is involved in the delivery of health care services. He, like the millions of hospital support-staff (and ancillary staff) around the world, is one of the people who makes the system, and the current set of health services, succeed or fail.

People can express their professional autonomy by non-performance of certain procedures. Perhaps the taxi driver's alleged action was an example of this, an expression of his choice not to be party to something he regarded as unacceptable. Is that any different from the fact that Catholic health care institutions do not provide abortions? You may like to think about the difference between not being party to something, and actively stopping such procedures from happening under someone else's purview.

Religious groups routinely adopt, and act on, positions on health issues. Consider, for instance, the following Roman Catholic Church position on AIDS health-education. The extract, from the St Vincent's *Bioethics Newsletter*, comments on a workshop on AIDS held by the St Vincent's Bioethics Centre, in Melbourne: 'The plenary sessions highlighted the urgent need for the Catholic community to respond to the inadequacy of the 'safe sex' approach to AIDS education, its need to integrate its services with those already existing in the wider community, its role as a witness to personal compassion as a remedy to the fear incipient in such a public health crisis and its leadership as the largest religious grouping in Australia.'[36]

There clearly is a difference between condoning an action and providing compassionate care for people affected by, or at risk from, that action. This is similar to the difference between, on the one hand, the obligation to provide care, and on the other, the obligation (in cases where clients have done something that we find abhorrent, or where we have ethical objections to the treatment they desire) to pass the responsibility for care on to others.

Health care workers occasionally come face to face with this difference. For instance, at the time of the Port Arthur massacre in Tasmania, the injured victims and the alleged gunman were brought for hospital treatment to the same emergency department. Workers dealt with the injured victims as well as the alleged perpetrator, all of whom were entitled to the best available care on offer. Those who felt that, if confronted with the responsibility of dealing with the alleged gunman, they could not place the best interests of the patient first, excluded themselves from the job of caring for the alleged gunman. A challenge to our willingness to care may be posed by our cultural, as well as our moral sense of good, as is discussed by Olsen in relation to nursing.[37]

Summary of key issues

- Community consultation and community expectations
- Institutional standards
- Beliefs and religion, as an overlay

Notes

1   H. Jonas, 'Philosophical Reflections on Experimenting with Human Subjects' *Daedalus*, vol. 98, no. 2, 1969, p. 245.

2   G. B. Ferngren, 'Roman Lay Attitudes Towards Medical Experimentation' *Bulletin of the History of Medicine*, Winter vol. 59, no. 4, 1985, p. 496.

3   B. M. Dickens, 'Issues in Preparing Ethical Guidelines for Epidemiological Studies', *Law, Medicine & Health Care*, vol. 19, no. 3–4, 1991, p. 183.

4   R. Nicholson, 'Bioethics Attacked in Germany' (editorial review), *Bulletin of Medical Ethics*, vol. 61, 1990, p. 22.

5   M. Douglas, 'Risk Acceptability According to the Social Sciences', *Social Research Perspectives—Occasional Reports on Current Topics*, Russell Sage Foundation, New York, 1985, p. 5.

6   M. S. Frankel, 'The Development of Policy Guidelines Governing Human Experimentation in the United States: A Case Study of Public Policy-Making for Science and Technology', *Ethics in Science & Medicine*, vol. 2, 1975, p. 46.

7   Staff reporters, 'Troubled transplant man throws in bad hand', *The Australian* Monday 5 February, 2001, p. 5.

8   R. Lovell, 'Ethics at the Growing Edge of Medicine—the Regulatory Side of Medical Research', *Australian Health Review*, vol. 9, no. 3, 1986, pp. 234–50.

9   C. A. Berglund, 'A Survey of Sydney Adults about the Conduct of Medical Research', *Australian Health Review*, vol. 17, no. 1, 1994, pp. 135–44.

10 I. Chalmers and W. A. Silverman, 'Professional and Public Double Standards on Clinical Experimentation', *Controlled Clinical Trials*, vol. 8, no. 4, 1987, pp. 390–1.

11 NHMRC, 'The National Health and Medical Research Council and Ethical Regulation—a Short History', *Australian Health Review*, vol. 9, no. 3, 1986, p. 236.

12 A. Campbell, 'Ethics in a bicultural context—a report from New Zealand', *Bioethics*, vol. 9, no. 2, 1995, pp. 149–54.

13 See, for example, A. Mulhall, 'Anthropology, Nursing and Midwifery: A Natural Alliance?', *International Journal of Nursing Studies*, vol. 33, no. 6, 1996, pp. 629–37.

14 J. S. Mill, 'On Liberty', in *Three Essays*, Oxford University Press, London, 1975, pp. 92–114.

15 H. Zwart, 'Rationing in the Netherlands: The Liberal and Communitarian Perspective', *Health Care Analysis*, vol. 1, 1993, pp. 53–6.

16 R. J. Sullivan, *Immanuel Kant's Moral Theory*, Cambridge University Press, Cambridge, 1989.

17 D. De Grazia, 'Moving Forward in Bioethical Theory: Theories, Cases, and Specified Principlism', *Journal of Medicine and Philosophy*, vol. 17, 1992, p. 525.

18 *National Health and Medical Research Council Act 1992* (Cwlth).

19 E. Dunne, 'Consultation, rapport, and collaboration: essential preliminary stages in research with urban Aboriginal groups', *Australian Journal of Primary Health Interchange*, vol. 6, no. 1, 2000, pp. 6–14.

20 P. Peel, 'Community participation in decision-making and service delivery', *Canberra Bulletin of Public Administration*, vol. 94, 1999, pp. 34–51.

21 Institute of Medicine (USA), *The AIDS Research Program of the National Institutes of Health*, National Academy Press, Washington DC, 1991, pp. 44, 45.

22 N. Gilmore, 'The Impact of AIDS on Drug Availability and Accessibility', *AIDS*, vol. 5, supplement no. 2, 1992, sections 253–62.

23 For instance, a dramatic increase in reporting of health issues has been demonstrated in the USA: R. C. Heussner Jr and M. E. Salmon, 'Where Medicine and Media Clash', *Minnesota Medicine*, vol. 72, no. 3, 1989, p. 141.

24 As proposed by V. Price and D. F. Roberts, 'Public Opinion Processes', in C. R. Berger and S. H. Chaffee (eds), *Handbook of Communication Science*, Sage, Newbury Park, California, 1987, pp. 784, 788.

25 NHMRC, *The Media and Public Health: A Discussion of the Role of the Media in Promoting the Health of the Public, Standing Subcommittee on Health Promotion and Education*, Sub-Committee on the Media and Health Promotion, Canberra, August 1984, p. 11.

26 N. Milio, 'The Press and Policy-Making: Clues for Creating a Health-Promoting Climate', *International Quarterly of Community Health Education*, vol. 10, no. 4, 1989–90, pp. 329–45.

27 C. A. Berglund, E. A. O'Brien, and A. G. Magney, 'Communication and Discussion of Health Research in the Press', platform paper presented at the Australasian and New Zealand Association for Medical Education Silver Anniversary Conference—Communication: Art and Science; Past and Future; Near and Far, 6–9 July 1997, Melbourne, pp. 25–33.

28 J. Walker, K. Lyall, and R. Hawes, 'Wooldridge Backs Inquiry on Guinea-Pig Babies', *The Australian*, 11 June 1997, pp. 1, 2; S. Dow, 'Trials and Terror: Medical Ethics Under the Microscope', *Sydney Morning Herald*, Saturday 14 June 1997, p. 35.

29 W. C. De Vries, 'The Physician, the Media, and the 'Spectacular' case', *Journal of the American Medical Association*, vol. 259, no. 6, 1988, p. 886.

30 'Nigerian woman resists deportation', *Africa News Service*, 21 November 2000, p. 1008325u3785.

31 G. W. Schneider and L. Snell, 'C.A.R.E.: an approach for teaching ethics in medicine', *Social Science & Medicine*, vol. 51, no. 10, 2000, pp. 1563–7.

32 T. Honderich (ed.), *The Oxford Companion to Philosophy*, Oxford University Press, New York, 1995, p. 761.

33 R. M. Veatch, *Cross Cultural Perspectives in Medical Ethics*, Jones and Bartlett Publishers, Boston, 1989.

34 J. Devereux, *Medical Law: Text, Cases and Materials*, Cavendish, Sydney, 1997, pp. 14–23.

35 K. Singh and G. L. Gan, 'An Asian Perspective on Euthanasia', *Australian Quarterly*, vol. 68, no. 3, 1996, p. 40.

36 St Vincent's *Bioethics Newsletter*, vol. 6, no. 4, 1988, p. 12.

37 D. P. Olsen, 'Populations Vulnerable to the Ethics of Caring', *Journal of Advanced Nursing*, vol. 18, 1993, pp. 1696–700.

8

Monitoring and education

Overview

- Peer standards and implementation
- Institutional standards and implementation
- Legal standards and ethics
- Self-reflection

This chapter concentrates on the way in which ethics standards come to be voiced in practice, and how ethics education occurs in the real world. The process of reflection on ethics is examined, as is the process of having standards set by others. The workings of ethics committees are used as a case study of how ethics is debated in particular forums. Readers are alerted to ways of keeping up to date with the, often regularly changing, standards that might affect them.

PEER STANDARDS AND IMPLEMENTATION

It is vital in professional practice to be aware of proper professional conduct, and of limits that should not be exceeded. You need to be vigilant in respect of both your own behaviour and the behaviour of others around you. You have a responsibility to work ethically, and to think about the broader ethics of the organisation for which you work. The themes, outlined in Chapter 1, of goals and duties, of aspiring to the highest practical standards of behaviour, and of abiding by rules are key factors in peer standards.

When harm could be caused by institutional or other professional behaviour, you may decide that the situation is serious enough to do something. You could try to educate your peers in an advisory way, or you could refer the matter to someone who can. Professional advice from colleagues, or such bodies as peer review committees and professional associations, may help. Take a look at your code of ethics; there is usually a clause about reporting unprofessional or unethical practices to the association that has drawn up the code. The association will usually have both informal and formal avenues for resolving such situations. Obligations to report unethical and/or unprofessional behaviour, and the methods for dealing with such reports, have the ultimate dual aims of protecting the public and protecting the profession's reputation.

Mentoring and continuing-education programs are an everyday part of professional life. Professional conferences and journals keep you up to date with standards and developing expectations, and with better ways of delivering service to match client expectations.

While professionals strive for excellence in care, mistakes sometimes occur, and can be serious. Medical errors are estimated to cause 270 deaths each day. A constructive discussion of adverse events and the development of a culture of open reporting to enable the discussion may be more effective in reducing future mistakes than a culture of blame and shame of individuals. However, open discussion and the gathering of information is constrained by the realities of legal process.[1]

The professional-standards committees of registration boards may investigate professional conduct. The complaints that prompt these inquiries can be made by anyone: the client, another member of the public, a fellow professional, or administrative staff. The powers of such committees are often set by the committees themselves, and once set, are enshrined in law; these laws are best understood with reference to a legal text.[2]

The following matters would be typical of registration-board inquiries: failure to attend in an emergency; lack of adequate knowledge, skill, judgement, or care; and cases where a practitioner's ability to provide care is impaired in some way. The treatment itself is a prominent source of complaint; for example, a complaint about an incorrect diagnosis or inappropriate treatment plan. The manner and politeness of the practitioner is also of great concern to many complainants.[3]

In Australia the exact operation of complaints processes varies between the states. In Victoria and New South Wales, complaints are made to the relevant ombudsman or the Health Care Complaints Commission. Each profession has its own way of hearing complaints, but most rely on the professional standards committees (or equivalent bodies) of registration bodies. Often, registration bodies are linked across states.[4] Nursing registration systems are often covered by parallel Acts in different states. Other health-profession registration systems range from mentoring by members of the association, to sanctions imposed by the association, to committee or judicial hearing.[5]

The emphasis of such monitoring or standards panels is to protect the public and to maintain the public trust in professional services. Public interest may be served by reprimanding the practitioner, educating the practitioner, and/or providing mentoring. The safety of the public is paramount. If a practitioner is thought to pose continued risk, the scope of his or her practice may be limited by restrictions imposed by the professional association. Serious matters that if proven may result in deregistration are considered by tribunals, with a presiding judge.

Committees can take the opportunity to pass their findings on to relevant professional associations, colleges, health departments, and hospitals, so that the lowered professional standards can be rectified and further unsatisfactory practice guarded against.

Registration boards are involved in proactive education, increased peer discussion forums for exchange of information, monitoring of performance, and support for higher risk practitioners, such as impaired practitioners, to contribute to standards maintenance and improvement. Summaries of activities can be found in the registration bodies' annual reports.[6] The impairment programs support impaired practitioners when they remain in practice. The programs necessarily include an element of treatment being provided for the practitioner, and possibly practice limits applied, so that the risk to the public is minimised. These programs can be applied at any time in a professional's career, for reasons of physical or psychological impairment. They rely to a great extent on the insight of the practitioner that further help is needed, should a change in their condition or a crisis occur, and a willingness of the practitioner to practise within safe limits. There may be a fundamental additional problem in applying these to students or professionals in periods of rapid learning and application of new skills. These people are in a process of skill acquisition rather than skill maintenance. The challenge is to support the individual, but anticipate when these periods of stress will be too much, so that patients remain safe at all times. For those practitioners, effective and alert mentors and supervisors are vital.

Some complainants find that official institutional or professional avenues are not sufficient to halt unsafe and/or unethical practices. Such complainants may face the uneasy dilemma of deciding whether to go outside the health care system and alert others to the practice. This is called whistleblowing. To 'blow a whistle' has had many colloquial meanings in the past. It has meant, variously, the whistle to stop work for a break (or smoko), the sounding of an alarm, or an alert to danger. Nowadays, whistleblowing has taken on the last of these meanings—an alert to danger. It is an alert, by a person, to the fact that an organisation, or someone within an organisation, is engaging in dangerous behaviour (or behaviour that is potentially dangerous). By definition, whistleblowing occurs when other internal alerts have failed. It is an alert to the world outside the organisation, a signal that an insider feels that public discussion is needed. The alert is made in the public interest. One definition of whistleblowing relied on by Vinten goes as follows: 'the unauthorised disclosure of information that an employee reasonably believes evidences the contravention of any law, rule or regulation, code of practice, or professional statement, or that invokes mismanagement, corruption, abuse of authority, or danger to public or worker health and safety'.[7]

It may take some time before the public becomes aware of the matter that a whistleblower is concerned about, as the example, described by Irene Blonder, on cervical cancer research in New Zealand shows.[8] In that research, women with early stage abnormalities of the cervix were examined over time, and no intervention was undertaken for some who subsequently progressed to stages of cervical cancer. When the colposcopist tried to raise his concerns within the medical profession, he encountered resistance, and at some later point decided to publish his concerns to promote discussion. Journalists pursued the matter and subsequently there was much discussion of it in both the popular and medical press. Finally, a government inquiry into the research was held. This research is discussed further in Chapter 9. Similarly, when the anaesthetist Stephen Bolsin tried to raise the issue of higher than normal mortality rates in children's heart surgery in one particular unit, and the lack of provision of those statistics to parents contemplating the surgery for their children, he encountered antagonism. Eventually, professional and public inquiries were convened, and his concerns supported. Bolsin moved to another country, feeling there would be limited career opportunities for him subsequently. He has told his story in a paper that is recommended tutorial reading on the process of professional concerns and speaking out, and should ideally be read along with subsequent commentaries and the Bristol inquiry report.[9]

Exercise 8.1 Professional concerns and trying to be heard

As a group, source Bolsin's article, and read what he says about his concerns and the process of trying to make his concerns heard.

Summarise the steps he went through to voice his concerns.

Note the different levels of recourse in his organisation and profession that he had available to him.

Can you suggest anything else that he could have tried?

This case was in the UK. Are there any differences in your own country?

What do you think of his eventual course of action in whistleblowing?

Many whistleblowers report that going outside their organisation and peer structure generated considerable resistance from their profession, and caused them personal hardship.[10] It is a difficult decision to make, and it should be considered carefully in respect of, first and foremost, the likely effect such an alert will have, and second, whether or not the problem might be constructively tackled at the peer or institution level, where it is occurring and where it impacts on clients.[11]

The crucial decisions in whistleblowing are:

- Is there an opportunity to make an internal report, rather than taking the complaint outside the profession or institution?

- Would whistleblowing educate the profession and the public about the problem?
- What are the risks involved?
- Is the harm sufficiently serious to warrant whistleblowing?
- What values are at stake?
- How timely would the alert be?
- What is the likely outcome of, on the one hand, pursuing the complaint internally, or on the other hand, whistleblowing?

INSTITUTIONAL STANDARDS AND IMPLEMENTATION

Informal peer monitoring is continual within institutions, as colleagues take the time to bounce ideas back and forth and discuss both past events and planned management. Formal institutional peer review is usually termed 'quality assurance', or simply 'QA'. Different hospitals set up different systems of QA, which although varying in process, share two basic elements: a process of overview, and a process whereby the relevant bodies are alerted to potential problems in standards of practice. Senior or junior members of staff can be called on to present their recent cases, and the cases are open for reflection and discussion. The aim is not to criticise individuals, but to ensure that high standards of care are maintained, and that all staff learn, from each other, ways to maintain that standard. Sometimes guidelines are developed from patterns of care that seem appropriate for particular conditions or types of clients.

There is a firmly held assumption that health care workers are striving to achieve the best for their clients, and are placing their clients' interests first. The ultimate goal of institutional standards is to streamline and clarify care so that the best care is delivered by the institutional team to the client.

As research ethics committees developed, they were increasingly asked to consider clinical (treatment) ethics issues in addition to their established role of considering research ethics. Some institutions have set up separate clinical ethics committees. More routinely, professionals resolve ethics issues within their own practice with team and peer assistance, but sometimes they seek ethics committee assistance, particularly when there is a complex issue involving a large team or conflicting views between carers and family. In the USA, committee involvement is more common, where ethics consultants are employed in large hospitals. They can have beepers and be on call for urgent consideration of ethics issues. In the UK, committees have developed relatively recently, and individual case consideration is possible.[12] Outside of the USA, ethics committees seem to concentrate more on policy formation to guide clinicians in complex cases in the future, rather than facilitate individual case decisions.[13] These are not necessarily dramatic issues. They could be as seemingly simple as when to allow care of a child to proceed without accompanying parents or guardians, or when to suggest a child be offered the opportunity to speak with their carer on their own. Or, how to ensure specific groups of clients make best use of available services, given cultural or physical limitations.

Exercise 8.2 From case decisions to policy

If you were working in a rehabilitation team, consider what assistance you would like to deal with the following case.

Try and identify issues that are case specific, and ones which could usefully be the subject of general policy.

You work in a rehabilitation team. A young man, Mr Y, aged 19 years, has come to see you. Mr Y's medical record shows that he has multiple health issues. He is slightly intellectually impaired, is on anti-epileptic medication, and has occasional rage outbursts. Recently, he was in a car with three friends, and was involved in an accident. At the time of the accident, one of his friends was riding on the roof of the car, and another was on the boot. The car was speeding on a dirt road, and rolled. Mr Y was inside the car, in the front passenger seat. He broke his leg so badly he had surgery, plates inserted, and is still on crutches. Mr Y's parents have rung you before the appointment. Apart from the lack of Mr Y's compliance with the physiotherapy suggested, they are worried about the risky behaviours, and want you to convince Mr Y to find new friends. Mr Y asks for your help in getting more independence from his family.

In identifying your issues, take the time to flick back through past chapters of this book, to refresh your memory on professional skill, resources and allocation, meeting and working with patients, developing and diminishing capacities, and so on. The scenario is quite a bit more complex than it seems on the surface.

When you have your issues identified, and divided into case specific and policy issues, try to solve one of each by group discussion.

For the case issue, role-play a process of consultation between relevant parties (after deciding who is relevant), and suggest a compromise between them.

For the policy issue, write a guiding principle, supported by ethics theory, that would help others in the future.

....

....

....

....

....

....

In research, ethics is formally considered at the institutional level, by the HREC (Human Research Ethics Committee), formerly called the Institutional Ethics Committee, or IEC. The concerns and workings of these committees are described in more detail in Chapter 9. All institutions that wish to be eligible for NHMRC funds must review the ethics of proposed research, regardless of whether that research is to be funded by NHMRC. In doing so, they refer to the principles expressed in the NHMRC's *National Statement on Ethical Conduct in Research Involving Humans*.[14] In this document, the required minimum composition of a committee is a chairperson, one layman, one laywoman, one minister of religion or person who performs a similar role in the community, one lawyer, at least one member with knowledge of and experience in the types of research considered regularly, and at least one member who has knowledge and experience in professional care and treatment of people. HRECs do not, strictly speaking, express institutional standards, because they remain independent from the institution, and their members are not, for the most part, employees of the institution. However, each committee sets the benchmark that must be applied in the institution that they serve.

HRECs do not often monitor research directly, but they do receive regular reports from researchers on their research, and on any adverse events that have accompanied this research, and can inspect research sites or records or interview participants if they wish either randomly or in response to concerns about research process or risks.[15] Professional associations are simply not resourced to directly monitor either. However, the strong professional responsibility enshrined in many professional codes effectively requires each professional to monitor the practice and behavioural standards of other professionals. Professionals have an obligation to report suspected unethical behaviour to the professional association.

LEGAL STANDARDS AND ETHICS

A sense of both the lower limits and the optimal levels (or ideals) of acceptable behaviour is introduced to you very early in this book, in Chapter 1. Many people would regard the minimum standard as being represented by law, and the upper, or optimal, level as represented by ethics. In short, law provides a minimum standard, while ethics acknowledges a minimum standard (which is not always the same as law) but strives for the maximal standard.[16] Both standards are fluid. Law is simply a reflection of what we regard as fair play and fair burden in our society.

Bentham is an example of a philosopher who has promoted a particular view of how ethics and law are related. An early utilitarian, Bentham espoused the principle of achieving the greatest good for the greatest number. The utility he concentrated on was felicity, or happiness, and the means to pursue it, Bentham thought, were reason and law. In brief, he thought that the stability of law would provide for a structure to achieve happiness. He felt that this fundamental aim of felicity should be recognised in law, and he set about suggesting legal and societal constructions that would do that. His concern was at a societal, and particularly a governmental level.[17] This was a grand plan to express societal goals and limits in a legal system. We in fact do use law to express societal expectations of professional behaviour.

Law is an empowering force in health care ethics. We use laws to give professions authority and mandate over their skill and the trade in that skill. Yet, we also use the law to constrain professionals if the standard is not met. As described previously, under legislation a complaints mechanism is available to anyone who feels that health care service standards, of whatever health profession, are not met. In New South Wales, the Health Care Complaints Commission is empowered by its own Act to investigate complaints, and then to refer the matter to the relevant professional panel or tribunal for consideration of whether the complaint is proven, and for a decision on penalties.

Laws relating to professional standards cover not only skill and competence, but also the manner in which service is provided and the character of the practitioner; in essence they cover the way that practitioners are ethical in their conduct of their work. These components of professional work were suggested to you in Chapter 1. The recognition of them in law is recognition of the intertwining of professional skill and proper conduct. Together, skill and ethics make an acceptable health care worker.

Broader societal expectations and standards are applied by law. This law is not limited to legislation passed by parliament and applied by either professional panels or tribunals. The laws governing such expectations and standards also come from the criminal and civil jurisdictions. In the criminal jurisdiction, laws about particular actions can limit what practitioners can become involved in. The most obvious examples are laws relating to abortion and those relating to the legality of euthanasia. Such laws are expressions of the lower limits of behaviour that society will tolerate. These limits are constantly debated by politicians, and can change. For instance, euthanasia was legal in the Northern Territory for a short time, until a debate in the Commonwealth parliament resulted in the law being overturned. Abortion and euthanasia are discussed more fully in Chapter 6.

The community, through the judiciary, can challenge the professions to change their ethics standards so that the professions stay in touch with community expectations. Judges are, broadly speaking, obliged by legal doctrine to follow previous decisions, called precedents. But they can, with reasoned legal arguments, come to a different conclusion and, therefore, a different decision. So, law is constantly evolving. The law acts as a safeguard for injured or 'wronged' clients, and as a message to other professionals that unless they apply certain standards in caring for their clients, they risk being sued.

Some legal systems virtually exclude civil action for damages, such as in New Zealand where there is a no-fault compensation scheme for injury. In these systems there are fears that this feature of the legal system has the effect of lowering standards of care. This fear has been analysed in a New Zealand legal study on complaints against doctors. The study found this fear to be unsubstantiated.[18]

Professionals need to be either up to date with the law, or find an avenue for being briefed on the latest developments in law. Ignorance of legal standards is not generally seen as an excuse for illegal behaviour, especially in criminal matters, even if the intentions behind the action were honourable.

SELF-REFLECTION

As you have worked your way through this book, you have been encouraged to undertake self-reflection. That is, you have been encouraged to reflect on what is important to you (and why), on what you should try to do (and why), on what you should not do, and on what you could do better.

In Chapter 1, you are asked to identify your own virtues, values, and important goals in your health care work. You are asked to acknowledge your skill limits, and the consequences if you were to overstep those bounds. You may be your own best safeguard in aspiring towards virtues and goals, and in not letting your standards drop too low. This process should continue throughout your professional life.

Take the time now to look back over all the reflective exercises you have done in previous chapters. As you browse through, consider how integral reflection is to the development of your skill and ethics, and in the application of your skill in an ethical manner.

Summary of key issues

- Continuing development and reflection
- Accountability to peers and society
- Law as a setter of societal limits

Notes

1   B. A. Liang, 'The adverse event of unaddressed medical error: identifying and filling the holes in the health-care and legal systems', *Journal of Law, Medicine & Ethics*, vol. 29, 2001, pp. 346–68, at p. 351.

2   A. Dix, M. Errington, K. Nicholson, and R. Powe, *Law for the Medical Profession in Australia*, 2nd edn, Butterworth Heinemann, Port Melbourne, 1996.

3 F. Faroque, 'Impolite Doctors Top List of Complaints', *The Age*, Saturday 7 December 1996, p. A8.

4 K. Breen, V. Plueckhahn, and S. Cordner, 'Medical Registration and Discipline', in *Ethics, Law & Medical Practice*, Allen & Unwin, St Leonards, 1997, pp. 77–99.

5 C. Thomson, 'Personnel', in *CCH Australian Health & Medical Law Reporter*, (looseleaf service), updated regularly, pp. 6–400.

6 Such as NSW Medical Board, *2002 Annual Report*, Gladesville, 2002.

7 G. Vinten, 'Whistle While you Work in the Health Related Professions?', *Journal of the Royal Society of Health*, vol. 114, no. 5, 1994, pp. 256–62.

8 I. Blonder, 'Blowing the Whistle', in M. Coady and S. Bloch, *Codes of Ethics and the Professions*, Melbourne University Press, Melbourne, 1996, pp. 166–90.

9 S. Bolsin, 'Professional misconduct: the Bristol case', *Medical Journal of Australia*, vol. 169, 1998, pp. 369–72; V. English, G. Roman-Critchley, J. Sheather, A. Sommerville, and G. Dehn, 'Would you "blow the whistle"?', *British Medical Journal*, vol. 325, 2002, p. 541; British Royal Infirmary Inquiry, *Learning from Bristol: the report of the public inquiry into children's heart surgery at the British Royal Infirmary*, London, Stationery Office, 2001.

10 K. J. Lennane, 'Whistleblowing: A Health Issue', *British Medical Journal*, vol. 307, 1993, pp. 667–70.

11 This is further discussed in C. Berglund, 'Thoughts Before Whistling', *Australian Health Review*, vol. 20, no. 4, 1997, pp. 5–12.

12 T. Hope and A. Slowther, 'Clinical ethics committee in the UK', *Bulletin of Medical Ethics*, 2002, vol. 178, pp. 13–15.

13 L. Doyal, 'Clinical ethics committees and the formulation of health care policy', *Journal of Medical Ethics*, vol. 27, Suppl. 1, 2001, pp. 144–9.

14 NHMRC, *National Statement on Ethical Conduct in Research Involving Humans*, Canberra, 1999.

15 As required by sections 2.33 to 2.38, supplementary note 1, principle 8, of the NHMRC, *National Statement on Ethical Conduct in Research Involving Humans*, Canberra, 1999.

16 See G. J. Annas, *Judging Medicine*, Humana Press, Clifton, New Jersey, 1988. Annas suggests that law is effectively QA and compensation for injury. See also G. Annas, *The Changing Landscape of Human Experimentation: From Nuremberg and Helsinki to AIDS and Cancer*, talk given at Grand Rounds, Royal Prince Alfred Hospital, Sydney, 7 August 1992.

17 T. Honderich (ed.), *The Oxford Companion to Philosophy*, Oxford University Press, New York, 1995, p. 85.

18 D. B. Collins, 'The Impact of No-Fault Compensation on the Regulation of Medical Practice in New Zealand', *Medicine & Law*, vol. 12, 1993, pp. 61–9.

9

And so to research

Overview

- Being a researcher and a carer
- Patient as research subject
- Prominent ethics concerns in research
- The Belmont principles
- Research ethics committees and submitting an ethics proposal

Professional health care workers are likely, at some stage, to undertake health research. This chapter is a practical guide to important ethical choices to be made in research. A checklist of prominent ethics concerns for major types of research projects is outlined. Readers are encouraged to express further ethics concerns themselves.

BEING A RESEARCHER AND A CARER

The general duty to do good and minimise harm is applicable to health research, just as it is to health care. While the benefits to the population that research may achieve are important, the first duty is to the client or research subject. Being a researcher and a carer is a delicate balance between ensuring ongoing trust in care relationships, and not exposing clients to unnecessary risks. Those who are both researchers and carers must come to understand their clients' conditions better at the same time as they are testing out options that may lead to better care for a wider class of people.

The importance of separating out research and caring roles was highlighted in the New Zealand cervical cancer experiments, discussed widely in the late 1980s.[1] (This case was noted, in Chapter 8, as an instance of whistleblowing.) In this research, women presented regularly for what they believed were thorough check-ups. They believed that they would be treated for any gynaecological conditions diagnosed in the course of these check-ups. They assumed that if they were not treated, then nothing was wrong with them.

The research was, in fact, to observe the development of pre-cancerous cervical cells. Many of the women progressed to cancer and died, while they were participating in the research. The research prompted debate about the institutional review standards that were applied when the hospital was considering the ethics of the research. This debate led to changes in the legal requirements laid down for the constitutions of New Zealand ethics committees.[2] Australia checked its own standards as a result, and institutions engaged in reflection on ethical safeguards.[3]

This long-term observation of the development of a condition is somewhat similar to the Tuskegee experiments, in which Black American men were observed, as their syphilis progressed without treatment. The observations continued even after treatment with penicillin became available.[4] Being a researcher brings with it responsibility to co-researchers (to ensure the integrity of the research), and to funding bodies. Care should be taken to declare potential conflicts of interests to supporting agencies. Divided loyalties to, on the one hand, a business that is funding the research, and on the other, caring institutions or patients, can be perceived by colleagues and the public as an unacceptable conflict of interest.

PATIENT AS RESEARCH SUBJECT

There are occasions when patients themselves push the bounds of treatment so that it effectively becomes research. They might have heard about a new treatment that they want to try, or there might be no known cure or treatment for their illness and they are willing to try anything.

This often happens when patients have a terminal condition, or a condition for which researchers and clinicians cannot offer an effective cure. There is well-established evidence that HIV/AIDS patients, for instance, consistently seek new and unproven treatments.[5] In effect, they force their carers to also become researchers. As there is a serious risk facing them, many people with HIV/AIDS might decide there is little distinction between research and treatment. As one AIDS community slogan states: 'A research trial is treatment too'.[6] The challenge posed to the drug-regulation system by making experimental drugs available is discussed in Chapter 2.

There is considerable responsibility placed on the individual health care worker in situations such as these. They still need to protect their patients from further harm, but when all available options have been tried, there is generally a willingness to let patients pursue more risky but as yet unproven treatments.[7] These treatments of 'last resort' do not have the same strict rules of drug regulation applied, so it need not always be in the context of a clinical trial if terminally ill patients wish to try something. A number of significant advances in cancer treatment have been developed as a result of aggressive treatments being tried by very ill people. Occasionally, world attention is focused on patients who choose radically new treatments; for example, in the mid 1990s, the so-called 'Baboon man' asked for baboon-marrow transplants to be given to him as a possible immune system boost. He was suffering from HIV/AIDS. At the time, the health care practitioner involved said that the only surprise was that the experimental treatment went so well. It did not make him better, but then, it did not make him worse either.[8]

At other times, carers will actually want their patients to try a new research protocol. The autonomous nature of the patient's decision is so important ethically, that it is routine for another health care researcher to recruit subjects. Patients can feel obliged to be participants if asked by their own carers. This feeling of obligation is termed 'dependency'.

PROMINENT ETHICS CONCERNS IN RESEARCH

When you conduct research with people, you are researching human participants. The following list is of some possible methods of researching health in human participants:

- accessing medical records
- asking questions in an interview or questionnaire
- doing a physical examination
- performing a blood test or taking a tissue sample
- giving an experimental treatment
- doing an experimental operation.

You may be able to think of more types of research. If you can, note them down. You may notice that the methods above are expressed in terms of what you do with the participants. That reflects the key ethics concern in research: what are research subjects being asked to do? This is where ethical reflection on research should start. You may also notice that as the list progresses, the level of invasiveness increases. Research subjects, health care workers, and the community are particularly concerned with how much invasiveness or intrusion research subjects are being asked to consent to.

You may be surprised that all of these methods are thought of as involving human participants. Even looking at medical records or analysing blood and tissue samples is thought of as researching people. In short, the people do not have to be right in front of you for your research to be thought of as having human participants.

A few general questions should start you on the way to ethical reflection on research that you may have conducted.
- *What was your research about?*
- *Were you skilled enough to undertake the research?*

- *Where did your research subjects come from?*
- *What did you ask your research subjects to do?*
- *How did the participants consent to the research?*
- *How was your research used?*
- *Was the process worth it, given the results?*

You could answer these questions for any research project that you undertake or that you see around you.

Exercise 9.1 Ethics analysis of research

As an exercise in applying these questions, take the time to look through a professional journal that is relevant to your profession. Many libraries have their recent journal copies displayed on reading shelves, and you can easily skim through a few to find a research article. Back copies are normally located in bound volumes on the library shelves. You could try visiting a university library, a hospital library, or a community library, which should all have a selection of health related journals.

A research article is one that explains the result of a research process, including the background of the research, the method of the research, what was found, and the researchers' interpretation of the findings.

When you answer each of the questions, make some notes on what you think the ethical significance of each issue is. Then, discuss your views with a friend or colleague.

The answer to each question has ethical significance, as is explained below.

What is the research about, and are you skilled enough to undertake it?

Research should have a purpose, a reason sufficient to justify the inconvenience or risk posed to the research participants. Researchers have a responsibility to care for research subjects, which includes being skilled enough to maximise care and minimise risk.

How are research subjects to be recruited, and what are they being asked to do?

The recruitment of research subjects involves questions of acceptable burden, and free choice, on the part of subjects, in their decision to participate. What research subjects are asked to do can determine the ethics of research: an ethical limit to the burden or risk to be borne by participants is always considered, but this limit can change depending on the importance of the research, and the endemic risks faced by the potential participant.

How are the research subjects being asked to consent?

The consent of research subjects is paramount, particularly as research is, by definition, not necessarily for their benefit—there is little room to justify paternalism.

For what purposes will the research be used and was the research worthwhile?

The likely use of the research determines both the importance of the research to the public, and the benefit for individual participants. Research can change how we think about best available treatment, or how we assess health, or it can consolidate what we already know. Practical use of research indicates that putting research subjects through the research has been worth it. Only once the process is understood and the results are known, can we really decide whether the research has been justified. The difficulty in terms of ethics is that this question has to be hypothetically answered before the research begins.

All the issues mentioned in relation to the above questions are inter-related. For instance, if a method is inappropriate because it does not fit the research purpose or produces erroneous results, the research could be seen as unethical, because (given the fact that no advancement in knowledge will occur) the inconvenience to the subjects is for no purpose. If the subjects were drawn from a vulnerable or dependent population, and the research was used to improve health care for the affluent only, we may decide that the research is unethical because it is unjust. More connections between these issues are explored below, within the context of a principlist examination.

THE BELMONT PRINCIPLES

The Belmont principles—beneficence, respect for persons, and justice—are used as tools here to further identify and examine key ethics concerns in research. As is suggested earlier in this book, the principles are useful as a shorthand way of checking that relevant moral concerns are taken into account. You should feel free to add your own specific ethics concerns to these principles.

Issues involving assessment of the risks and benefits to individuals can be thought of as coming under the principle of beneficence; issues surrounding personal autonomy as being under the principle of respect for persons; and issues of the benefits and burdens to society in general as coming under the principle of justice. This categorisation of issues is consistent with the Belmont Report's suggestions for the use of these principles.[9] The principles should all be considered in any research situation. That is because some issues relate to more than one principle—there can be conflicting ethical concerns in research practice, as in any health practice.

Beneficence

The maxim 'do no harm', a major element of beneficence, is critical in research. This is because it is not always possible to achieve the other element of beneficence—the injunction to 'do good'—for each research participant. This is in spite of the future benefits to others, benefits which are frequently claimed as a justification for research.

An honest appraisal of what, and how much, benefit is likely from the research is needed. This benefit constitutes both the private and public interest in conducting the research, because some benefit may be to the individual participant, either in the course of the research or shortly thereafter, and some benefit may be to the community in the future. You can ask yourself the following question: What purpose does this research serve?

A risk assessment is a crucial first step in avoiding harm. The amount of risk acceptable (and by whom), and how that risk is assessed is of ethical concern. Even though some studies suggest that risk to research participants is low in most cases, any risk potentially violates the maxim 'do no harm'.[10] That means that all risk, even if minimal, should be explicitly acknowledged and documented.

After acknowledging risk, the next step is to assess whether that risk is acceptable. If the participant is already facing some sort of risk because, for example, he or she is suffering from an illness, this can make a difference to the ethical acceptability of research. If the proposal aims, ultimately, to reduce that risk, then this affects the risk–benefit assessment. The World Medical Association's Declaration of Helsinki makes use of the distinction between therapeutic and non-therapeutic research, in assessing acceptable risk (this distinction and its implications for consent are discussed in Chapter 5). This Declaration states that greater risk is acceptable if the research is therapeutic and may do good to individuals. The benefits and harms of a potential therapeutic treatment are weighed against the benefits and harms of treatments already available.[11] The level of risk acceptable in non-therapeutic research is lower. Under the Declaration of Helsinki, research must be discontinued if harm may be caused to the participant.[12] An obligation to benefit and to do no harm is important in both therapeutic and non-therapeutic research. As the researcher's ability to fulfil the 'do good' maxim diminishes, his or her responsibility to fulfil the 'do no harm' maxim increases correspondingly. Ethics committees increasingly weigh up the 'value' of proposed research and the risk it entails.[13]

Risk can, of course, be difficult to assess, especially in procedures that have not been used before. In assessing risk in such situations, it may be useful to rely on similar research conducted previously on animals or very early approximations to human use (for example, in vitro examination of blood or tissue response). A high level of clinical and scientific judgement is needed to make this risk assessment. The acceptability of risk is necessarily a value judgement. You, as a researcher, decide what you are prepared to ask people to undertake. Ethics committees make a similar judgement before research proceeds. Participants decide whether they are prepared to participate, and they take on those risks, for potential benefit to themselves or/and others.

The concern in all research is that some invasive procedure, whether physical or non-physical, may be performed on a participant. In medical research, this invasion is likely to be to the physical integrity of the person, but in non-medical research, this invasion is more likely to be to the psychological integrity of the person. Both physical and psychological integrity are essential to the well-being of the individual, and must be protected. Consistent with that concern is a commitment by the researcher to stop the research if the risk to this integrity becomes too great.

Respect for persons

The principle of 'respect for persons' seeks to ensure that an individual's wishes are respected, even if they differ from those of the researcher, or from those expected of the individual by the researcher. Each potential participant should be given the opportunity to express their wishes before being included in the research, and throughout the research process. Broadly, the principle implies respect for rights, wishes, and individuality of the participant. Allowing for informed consent to research, and maintaining confidentiality of data are processes that uphold the dignity and individuality of research participants.

The fundamental ethical standard in research is that people should take part of their own free will. This is expressed in the United Nations Covenant on Civil and Political Rights as follows: 'no one shall be subjected without his free consent to medical or scientific experimentation'.[14] It is echoed in all research ethics codes. In order to uphold the integrity of the consent process, individuals who have the capacity to make decisions about research participation should be allowed to do so. They should also be free to withdraw at any time.

Apart from competency to make decisions, the capacity for autonomous decision making also requires an environment that is free of coercion. If the environment is not free of coercion, a request for participation may not be ethical. This means that refusal to consent should not lead to any detriment (other than the agreed-upon risks of the research) or loss of standing for the patient. A non-coercive environment also means that there should be no such implied threat either. Informed consent as a health care process is examined in Chapter 3.

Control over personal information is a fundamental extension of the principle of 'respect for persons'. It means giving an individual control over information about him or her—not just control over their own physical self, which is often protected by consent. Confidentiality of information implies that personal information should be held in confidence, and should not be included in any further research or made available for other purposes, unless the individual whom the information is about gives consent. Confidentiality obligations are tested in research that uses information that is already stored for another purpose (such as medical records) and in research that involves collecting information that may be useful for another purpose. Use of personal information for purposes other than those consented to requires that there is sufficient public interest in those further purposes. In relation to Commonwealth research, ethics committees are, ultimately, the only bodies that can decide this (under the provisions of the *Privacy Act*), and they are increasingly choosing to apply *Privacy Act* standards in other public and private jurisdictions. This is explored more fully in Chapter 4.

Ideally, research participants should be aware of the research process, as it progresses from start to finish. This includes being informed of the results of the research, so that they may learn from it and can maximise the benefit or minimise the potential harm, of the research for their own lives. To use people as subjects, but not inform them of the results (if they wish to know the results) could seem exploitative.

A further area in which there is potential for exploitation is payment. The question of how much, if at all, to pay research subjects is difficult to resolve, and depends ultimately on the population from which research subjects will be chosen. Some compensation for participation is preferable, but it should not be so large as to amount to coercion to participate. Many researchers use a model of 'compensation for time'—in the form of issuing travel taxi vouchers, and providing lunch vouchers for the day of the research—rather than monetary payment, which could induce low-income earners or unemployed people to take part in risky research for the money. This would effectively exploit that less affluent section of the population for the benefit of the whole population.

Justice

The principle of justice involves considering the fair distribution of the benefits and burdens of research within society. To achieve that, the duty of professionals to conduct research and to advance knowledge so that society may benefit needs to be acknowledged. The advancement of knowledge cannot be at the expense of the individual patient or research subject, so effectively, concerns of beneficence and respect for persons take precedence. Research should not be regarded as ethical, no matter how great the community benefit, if individuals suffer too greatly in the conduct of that research. This concern over the suffering of research subjects is at the heart of criticisms of war-time experiments conducted by the Nazis during World War Two, and is a constant concern where underprivileged or institutionalised participants are used for research that is designed for the benefit of privileged or non-institutionalised persons.

You should note that, in theoretical terms, placing beneficence and respect for persons over justice makes explicit the distinction between, on the one hand, the good for the individual, and on the other, the common good. This distinction is often a source of confusion when applying the principles of beneficence and justice.[15] Economic writers may challenge the primacy of other principles over justice, preferring to set societal objectives (such as economic growth), which can be used to implement beneficence and respect for persons.[16]

On a practical level, you need to assess what the social benefits and burdens of the research are, assess who or which groups bear the burden of research, and determine who or which groups potentially benefit from the research. Only then can a decision on the acceptability of the research be made.

The sharing of knowledge and the dissemination of information gained from research is an element of the duty to society to conduct research so that benefits and burdens are distributed more knowledgeably and fairly within society. If you are conducting research, you should write up and present your results accurately, noting its pitfalls as well as its successes. Your findings and your description of the research should be made publicly available; for example, at conferences, professional forums, or professional journals. It is also advisable to make this information available in a form that can be accessed by the community.

Dissemination of knowledge saves the same burden of risk being placed on future prospective research participants. It maximises the potential benefits of research: disseminating the knowledge gained from the research allows others to move further on the basis of your results, instead of repeating the research because they are not aware of your results (or failing to offer the best available treatment because they are not aware of your research results).

In summary, the key ethics points for researchers are:
- beneficence
- assessment of the benefits of the research
- assessment of the risks of the research
- weighing risk against benefit
- respect for persons
- informed consent from research subjects
- research subjects should be free to withdraw from the research
- confidentiality
- informing research subjects of results

- paying/compensating research subjects
- justice
- advancement of knowledge for the benefit of society
- assessment of distribution of benefit
- assessment of distribution of burden
- fair balance of benefit and burden
- sharing of knowledge and dissemination of results.

RESEARCH ETHICS COMMITTEES AND SUBMITTING AN ETHICS PROPOSAL

Ethics committees provide an opportunity for professional, institutional, and community concerns about clinical practice and research practice to be discussed and decided on. The committees provide useful referral processes for clinicians, and they are essential for researchers, who need their approval before they can conduct research. More on clinical ethics committees is included in Chapter 8.

There can be some confusion about how to refer to ethics committees. In Australia, committees that consider research ethics are called human research ethics committees (HRECs) but prior to 1999 were called institutional ethics committees (IECs). The same committees are called 'research ethics committees' in the United Kingdom, and 'institutional review boards' in the USA. In Australia committees that consider clinical treatment ethics are called clinical ethics committees, but they are called IECs in the USA. This section is headed 'research ethics committees', because the term 'research' denotes the function of the committees. In Australia, the key ethics standard to consider when submitting a research proposal to an ethics committee, is the NHMRC *National Statement on Ethical Conduct in Research Involving Humans*. This standard is important because all HRECs are obliged to consider research in the light of the principles it promotes. It is now accompanied by a lengthy manual, designed to assist researchers and ethics committee members to apply the principles in the Statement.[17] You can access the Statement on the internet, at <www.nhmrc.gov.au>, and you should do so if you are planning to conduct any research.

Similar statements all around the world have been developed in the interests of protecting human subjects and also maintaining the progress of understanding through medical research. The statements are designed to ensure that unethical research, such as that examined in the Nuremberg trials, does not occur again. The Nuremberg trials examined, among other war crimes, medical research conducted on Nazi-held prisoners of war. Those responsible for the experiments were put on trial and were, ultimately, convicted of having committed crimes against humanity. The experiments included sterilisations, placing people in freezing conditions to observe the effect on their body, infecting people with typhus to observe the reaction, and even killing so that the body could be dissected as a specimen. The resulting Nuremberg Code, setting out principles of how to deal with research subjects with respect and preserving their dignity, forms a vivid historical backdrop to many subsequent discussions of the ethics of research with human participants.[18]

The World Medical Association's Declaration of Helsinki is the base document of many research guidelines that have been developed. This is routinely discussed and updated at assembly meetings, but retains its name of Helsinki, as that was the city where the meeting was held that approved the early version of the Declaration. The balance of maintaining research in different contexts was under discussion for amendment in 2003 and 2004, as discussed in Chapter 2.[19] The background to the issue is that when new treatments are being trialed, there is most commonly (but not always) a comparison group, who do not receive the new treatment. This is so that the effects of the trial treatment on the research participants can be compared and evaluated against others with similar conditions, and not just against changes in condition of the human participants who are receiving the treatment. This forms a more reliable comparison, and is the standard approach in quantitative research studies.[20] Traditionally, placebo groups were the comparison, and those in the placebo group did not receive treatment of any kind. Now, however, the norm is that the best proven and available treatment is given to those in the comparison group, so they are no worse off than if they were not in a research trial. The effect of the new treatment can then also be compared to how people progress if they received the standard treatment of the day. In the developing world, the difficulty is that the best proven treatment may simply not be affordable or available to people. It is a difficult ethical quandary for researchers who want to help and fulfil their duty to take part in improving medical care and treatment, to decide what their responsibilities are to research subjects in countries where basic care is not as good, or lacks many choices available to similar research subjects in the developed world. The WMA may address this by limiting professional responsibility to pursuing locally available best available treatment for the participants, both during and after the conclusion of the trial, although the proposed amendment is highly controversial and has prompted heated discussion.

So, reference to professional codes, national guidelines, and international standards should be routine for researchers who are planning research. These are designed to help researchers conduct research ethically, and should be referred to by professionals in addition to seeking peer deliberation and discussion of issues. Ethics committees have an educative function, as well as a gate-keeping role. They can be asked for advice when researchers face difficult issues.

If you are preparing to submit your research proposal, first contact your ethics committee and ask them the following questions:
• Is there a pro-forma for submission?

- When does the committee meet?
- What is the deadline for your submission to be included in the agenda for the next meeting?

It is common practice for proposal deadlines to be one or two weeks before the meeting date. This allows time for agendas to be prepared; for the committee to identify if the proposal is missing any information (and to ask for this missing information); and to make copies of the proposal and distribute these to the ethics committee members. The members read the proposals before they meet, and they are expected to give each proposal due consideration.

You, as a researcher, need to be aware of that review and reflection process, and give it the time it deserves. There may be administrative requirements particular to your ethics committee: for example, your committee may require you to submit multiple copies of the proposal. Find out these administrative details early on, preferably well ahead of the deadline for proposal submission, so that you do not miss the deadline for the meeting. Committees may only meet four times a year. You need to be careful that you do not unduly delay the granting of ethics committee approval.

Exercise 9.2 A proposal for consideration

Try this group discussion exercise. Allocate roles to people along the lines of ethics committee composition. You will remember that committees have as a minimum, a chairperson, two laypeople, a minister of religion or community elder, a lawyer, a researcher in the relevant field, and a clinician from any of a variety of health professions. Various ages are commonly sought for this membership.

A community health fund has promised funding for a trial of a new treatment of eye infection, in a remote area, populated largely by indigenous people. The researchers plan to provide refrigeration equipment for the duration of the trial which is needed for the medicine and preparations, as this is lacking in the area routinely. The research will extend over a two-year period. People of all ages who attend the monthly community health clinic, and who are diagnosed by the community health nurse as having a particular type of eye infection, will be offered the chance to take part in the research. Half (randomly assigned on the basis of random numbers allocated for the sequence in which they attend) will be asked to follow the routine advice given, and the other half will be offered the new treatment regime. Researchers will follow-up all people at monthly intervals, and serious deterioration in any participants will trigger a new assessment of treatment requirements. This assessment that would be offered would take place in a community base hospital. Transportation for the assessment would be arranged by the research team. Subsequent different treatment advice and treatment arrangements if they needed to withdraw from the research would be the responsibility of the individual and community.

As a committee, consider the proposal. Be guided by an example of a research guideline, such as the NHMRC *National Statement*, and a general ethics guideline, such as your profession's code of ethics.

Once research is underway, the responsibility for monitoring the ethical conduct of it is shared: the researcher continues to reflect on the ethical dimensions of the process, as do their peers, the institution, the ethics committee, the funders, the participants, and the community. Ethics committees can monitor and audit actively all research within their institutions, regardless of funding source, and in some countries, government funded offices undertake this responsibility for publicly funded research. For instance, public offices such as the US Office of Research Integrity, set guidelines for research conduct and assessing alleged research misconduct in publicly funded research. Information can be given to them by any complainants. Routine random audits can also be undertaken to check for study teams who disregard discrepant data, or data that doesn't 'fit' their hoped for outcome, and generally check the integrity of data files and patient records. Urgent investigations are conducted if there is an 'immediate public health hazard'.[21]

Exercise 9.3 Monitoring and investigation

Try this tutorial exercise, imagining that you have to investigate an allegation about research misconduct, made by a research participant, Patient B.

A new treatment is being trialed for the control of a chronic and debilitating condition, and Patient A is a close friend of Patient B. Although random allocations are meant to occur, Patient A apparently asked to be assigned to the treatment group after realising that the medication she was assigned was no different to that which she had been taking for some time in the context of routine treatment. She had taken the medication she was given for the research trial to an independent lab and asked that it be analysed. It was three weeks after the trial had started, but she managed to change groups, and all of her data was allegedly transferred to the 'treatment' group for inclusion in that analysis. Patient B is disgruntled that she may be on the comparison group treatment, and has been told she cannot be told which group she is in, and in any case, cannot change groups.

Or, alternatively, consider an allegation made by a junior member of a research team, in a large multi-institutional trial, that the published findings differ to that in the research records.

Consider what sort of evidence would need to be collected in order to investigate the allegations.

If proven, what action do you think should be taken in regards to:

• the participants, if any

....

....

....

....

....

....

....

• the investigators

....

....

....

....

....

....

....

• the institution

....

....

....

....

....

....

Look up the ORI website, at <www.ori.hhs.gov>, to see if its summaries of investigations match your proposed process of investigation. Its 'evidence' records may help too. The basic process is to check facts, assuming there is a consent from research participants for the records to be available for audit, and interpret them with the assistance of knowledgeable peers.

Summary of key issues

- Responsibilities to care and to advance knowledge
- Ethics as part of research design
- Ethics as part of research process
- Administrative requirements
- Regulations

Notes

1 S. Coney, *The Unfortunate Experiment: The Full Story Behind the Inquiry into Cervical Cancer Treatment*, Penguin, Auckland, 1988.

2 G. Gillett, 'The New Ethical Committees: Their Nature and Role', *New Zealand Medical Journal*, vol. 102, 1989, pp. 314–15.

3 P. M. McNeill, 'The Implications for Australia of the New Zealand Report of the Cervical Cancer Inquiry: No Cause for Complacency', *Medical Journal of Australia*, vol. 150, 1989, pp. 264–96.

4 J. H. Jones, *Bad Blood: The Tuskegee Syphilis Experiment*, Free Press, New York, 1981.

5 C. Levine, N. N. Dubler, and R. J. Levine, 'Building a New Consensus: Ethical Principles and Policies for Clinical Research on HIV/AIDS', *IRB: A Review of Human Subjects Research*, vol. 13, nos 1–2, 1991, pp. 1–17.

6 G. Annas, 'The Changing Landscape of Human Experimentation: From Nuremberg and Helsinki to AIDS and Cancer', talk given at Grand Rounds, Royal Prince Alfred Hospital, Sydney, 7 August 1992.

7 For instance, J. Oliver and D. J. Webb, 'Sildenafil for "blue babies". Such unlicensed drug use might be justified as last resort', *British Medical Journal*, vol. 325, no. 7373, 2002, p. 1174.

8 Associated Press, 'Baboon Man Out of Hospital', *Weekend Australian*, 6–7 January 1996, p. 11; 'Baboon Marrow Fails to Boost AIDS Patient', *The Australian*, 9 February 1996, p. 9.

9 United States Department of Health, Education, and Welfare, *Ethical Principles and Guidelines for the Protection of Human Subjects of Research* (the Belmont Report), DHEW publication no. OS 78–0012, United States Department of Health, Education and Welfare, Washington DC, 1978.

10 R. J. Levine, *Ethics and Regulation of Clinical Research*, Urban & Schwarzenberg, Baltimore and Munich, 1986, p. 39.

11 World Medical Association, Principle 11(2), Declaration of Helsinki 1964, as revised at the 35th World Medical Assembly, Venice 1983, World Medical Association, New York.

12 World Medical Association, Principle 111(3).

13 D. J. Cassarett, J. H. T. Karlawish, and J. D. Moreno, 'A taxonomy of value in clinical research', *IRB: Ethics & human research*, vol. 24, no. 6, 2002, pp. 1–6.

14 United Nations Covenant on Civil and Political Rights, in M. J. Bossuyt, *Guide to the 'Travaux Preparatoires' of the International Covenant on Civil and Political Rights*, Martinus Nijhoff Publishers, Dordrecht, 1987.

15 R. M. Veatch, 'Justice in Health Care: The Contribution of Pellegrino', *Journal of Medicine and Philosophy*, vol. 15, 1990, p. 277.

16 G. H. Mooney, E. M. Russell, and R. D. Weir, *Choices for Health Care: A Practical Introduction to the Economics of Health Provision*, 2nd edn, Macmillan, London, 1986, pp. 48, 49, 55.

17 National Health and Medical Research Council, *National Statement on Ethical Conduct in Research Involving Humans*, Canberra, 1999; NHMRC *Human Research Ethics Handbook: Commentary on the National Statement on Ethical Conduct in Research Involving Humans*, Canberra, Ausinfo, 2002.

18 S. F. Spicker, I. Alon, A. de Vries, and H. T. Englehardt (eds), *The use of human beings in research: with special reference to clinical trials*, Kluwer Academic Publishers, Boston, 1988.

19 World Medical Association, 'WMA to continue discussion on Declaration of Helsinki', Press release, 14 September 2003, at <http://www.wma.net>.

20 C. A. Berglund (ed.), *Health research*, Oxford University Press, Melbourne, 2001.

21 Department of Health and Human Services (DHHS), *Guidelines for assessing possible research misconduct in clinical research and clinical trials*, DHHS, Rockville, MD, USA, 2001.

10

Ethics theories

Overview

- Absolutism/deontology
- Consequentialism/utilitarianism
- Proportionism
- Communitarianism
- Libertarianism
- Principlist frameworks
- Cases to ponder
- A guide to further reading

Key theorists are discussed and their theories applied to case studies to contrast the arguments that might be advanced under each theory or framework. Contemporary dilemmas in health care relationships and in the system of health care are used to highlight differences between theoretical arguments. Readers are encouraged to nominate which theories they are most comfortable with, and to reflect on their own values, which they are asked to define in Chapter 1, in order to understand why they would choose particular theories over others. This chapter explores the choice that must be made when confronting a dilemma about which values to emphasise.

ABSOLUTISM/DEONTOLOGY

Deontology works with the notion that there are certain absolute rules that must be followed, or upheld, regardless of the consequences. It classifies acts according to whether they must be done (because they are necessary to uphold a particular rule or rules), or are wrong (and therefore, must not be done). The rules are commonly thought to be handed down from God, such as the rule of sanctity of life. The rules translate into duties.

An example of the way in which rules translate into duties is included in Chapter 1. The moral importance of acting and not acting was the subject of an exercise in Chapter 3, in which you were asked to decide which protagonist in the story, Alex or Alice, was responsible for the harm that befell their father.

The 'doctrine of double effect', a classic deontological tool, is covered in Chapter 3. The responsibility for something bad occurring, even though a good was aimed for, is a key issue for health care workers.

The question of what constitutes personhood (and life) is addressed in Chapter 6. As the discussion in that chapter shows, deontological positions are prominent in this debate over the defining characteristics of personhood and life. The discussion contrasts these deontological positions with outcome-based positions, particularly in relation to the creation, genetic manipulation, and ending of life.

Deontology is in direct opposition to relativism, in which the question of what to do is defined not in reference to strict rules, but in reference to the relevant boundaries for that context or culture.

CONSEQUENTIALISM/UTILITARIANISM

Under consequentialist or utilitarian theories, which are teleological, the 'right' thing to do is that which maximises the good. The outcome of an action is what is ethically important. The greatest good for the greatest number is pursued, whether that good is a specific utility, felicity, or happiness.

These utilitarian assumptions are discussed in Chapter 2. Under utilitarianism, the question of how to share a limited good is often one of how to maximise distribution. It is possible to reject such utilitarian assumptions when making ethical decisions, as did those ethicists responding to the hypothetical scenario on predictive cancer testing, discussed in Chapter 2.

Peter Singer's view on obligations to care and even to work in some danger are described in Chapter 3. In his framework, one's own interests do not necessarily receive priority if the greatest good for the greatest number is the prime consideration in the issue at hand.

To look at the effect of manipulation of life, as was done in the case of Marissa and Anissa Ayala, discussed in Chapter 6, is to acknowledge the fact that ethically problematic decisions affect not only the individuals immediately concerned, but also whole communities.

PROPORTIONISM

Proportionism acknowledges rules and values, but does not regard them as universal. It is quite a pragmatic theory, which, without using binding principles as a guide, takes into account the human nature of the person, the situation, and the intention behind the person's actions. A broad idea of good is aimed for.

Doing the best one can is a common pragmatic approach to ethics. The proportionist would require that best is pursued in full knowledge of the ethical choices and practical alternatives.

Proportionism is essentially a compromise between the extremes of absolutism and relativism. Relativism, and in particular the work of the philosopher Harman, is mentioned in Chapter 1, as an example of an approach to the search for minimum acceptable standards that is often conducted when two groups differ on the appropriate course of action in treatment.

Relativism is not compatible with deontology, in which rules are universally applied, but it can be used in combination with other moral theories, such as utilitarianism or communitarianism. Relativism takes note of the rules or values that are appropriate for the context in which decisions are made.

Casuistry is also a pragmatic addition to ethics. It emphasises the importance of understanding value-laden decisions in their appropriate factual context and culture.[1] Legal reasoning, such as is discussed in Chapter 3, on informed consent, is very close to casuistry. It starts with the facts and context, and relates that to precedent. Precedent is law derived from previous decisions in cases involving the same or similar circumstances. To apply precedent in a legal context is to use a type of case-based legal decision making that applies certain legal principles derived from an accumulated history of case law to the particular facts of the dispute. Each new case tests whether the same precedent applies, given the slightly varied facts and circumstances.

COMMUNITARIANISM

Communitarianism places the community at the centre of a value system and its corresponding ethical analysis. While the individual members are acknowledged, it is the good of the community, its goals, and the threats it faces that are the key considerations. Communal and public goods are emphasised, and community views must be sought to unravel difficult issues.

The process of seeking and acknowledging community views has been discussed throughout this book. In Chapter 1, a comment by the former Director-General of WHO, Dr Nakajima, is included to show that professional ethics takes place within a community context, which implies that values of the community should be respected.

Chapter 3 discusses the fact that there are many different community values in relation to informed consent. The processes that make community views on ethics known are outlined in Chapter 7.

LIBERTARIANISM

Libertarianism places the personal freedom of the individual at the centre of analysis. That freedom is claimed as a right, unless there is sufficient reason to limit it. Patient freedom and autonomy is explored in Chapter 3.

J. S. Mill has been referred to throughout the book as a libertarian (a philosophy closely related to liberalism) philosopher. His thesis *On Liberty* has been used to decide when a person's liberty can be infringed, such as in the mandatory HIV testing exercise in Chapter 4. The only acceptable reasons for limiting liberty are if a serious and imminent risk is posed to another individual, or if the fabric of society is threatened. These reasons are used, at strategic points in this book, to explore the health care worker's role in fostering self-determination and being aware of similar rights to liberty held by others. Max Charlesworth was mentioned, in Chapter 3, as a modern libertarian writer.

PRINCIPLIST FRAMEWORKS

Principlist frameworks for decision making are a modern phenomenon. They are summarising tools that use shorthand principles that capture the obligations and aspirations of health care workers. These frameworks are a facilitative naming of principles, and as such, some thought needs to be applied in situations where the principles conflict.

Different principlist frameworks are described in Chapter 1, which contrasts those of Beauchamp and Childress—beneficence, non-maleficence, autonomy, and justice—with Gillon's principles (respect for autonomy, beneficence, non-maleficence, and justice). Chapter 1 uses the principles of Beauchamp and Childress as a tool to summarise issues in a vignette on general practice. They are also an essential part of the exercise requiring you to summarise your code of ethics. In Chapter 9 the Belmont principles of beneficence, respect for persons, and justice, are also used to highlight key ethics concerns in health care research.

These principles can be shown to be compatible with diverse ethical theories, as is shown in Chapter 1. It may be that, in a situation in which the principles are in conflict, different theories would prioritise the principles quite differently. For instance, while libertarianism's central value—individual freedom—emphasises autonomy, communitarianism's concern to achieve good for all (in a fair manner) emphasises justice. Drawing the line at harm that is unacceptable (even when the patient has indicated a willingness to be harmed, or there is a good that must be promoted) emphasises beneficence. Because the principles used in principlist frameworks are summarising principles, they should not be used alone. You can use a principlist approach in combination with any of the ethical theories outlined above.

CASES TO PONDER

The reflective exercises that you have been asked to do throughout this book are intended to galvanise you towards your own preferred ethical theory. Look back to the reflective exercises in Chapter 1. What you value and what you aim for, as a person and a health care worker, is central to your choice of ethics theory. Is your predominant aim to respect others' choices, or do you feel that doing the right and dutiful thing, with reference to carefully prescribed rules, is preferable? Your own ethical reflection is a continuing process that is only just beginning. As it develops, it will be moulded and tested by the challenges you will face in your work as a health care practitioner.

Now, you might like to consider the following few case studies. After each is set out, the key aspects that might be focused on under different theories are explained. It is up to you to ponder the key elements and think about how a solution to each problem might be arrived at. As you think, turn back through the book and re-read sections that you feel will become crucial in your argument.

Exercise 10.1 Multiple issues

CASE ONE

When you first met Ms Tan, she was 14. She has a slight mobility disability, from a congenital spinal problem, and is mildly intellectually disabled. With the aid of an interpreter (English is her second language), you arrived at a course of treatment and management for her recently diagnosed asthma, in close consultation with her other health care workers and her parents. Now, three years later, Ms Tan returns. She has left school, is working part-time, and has more ambitious life priorities, in keeping with a young adult. She asks for your help in continued treatment, but also in getting more independence from her family. She feels that they closet her because of her medical problems.

Patients rarely have just one medical or health concern. Their social context is also complex. How you define 'health' will lay the foundation for your reaction to this case with Ms Tan. You should first consider whether your definition of health is as broad as WHO's, which includes the physical, social, and mental aspects of life. The definition of health, and the good to aim for as a health care worker, is a central focus of Chapters 2 and 3.

Deontological theory would emphasise the duties owed to Ms Tan as an individual, especially the duty to further good for her and to limit harm coming to her, particularly intentional harm. There may be some rules that would preclude doing what she asks; for example, you might think that the process is fundamentally wrong.

If you adhere to the ethical theories that place most weight on patient autonomy, such as libertarianism, upholding Ms Tan's choices will be important to you, even if you do not agree with them. You will be concerned to establish that Ms Tan is competent to make certain relevant decisions and life choices. The issue of competence is covered in Chapter 5.

Ms Tan's cultural and family contexts are especially relevant in proportionism and communitarianism. Both theories balance goals, such as life and health goals, with individual variation and choice in relation to these goals, according to cultural and societal limits.

The question of whether allowing the choices she wants to make will result in good for her, her family, and society is a key factor in utilitarianism. This is because the good that is aimed for has a societal context also; that is, it has ramifications beyond Ms Tan as an individual.

So, while all theories rely on an obligation to care on the part of the health worker, they give startlingly different reasons for the existence of that obligation.

Exercise 10.2 Coordinating choices

CASE TWO

You are involved in a coordinated-care program, in conjunction with many different health care providers in your local area. The money available for care is controlled by a central coordinator, in this case a nurse, and the money is hypothetically capped for each chronic health problem. Your client, Mr Helm, is in his mid-forties and has many complex medical problems resulting from a car accident that happened five years previously. This accident left him with internal injuries. A new drug has just finished being tested, and has been registered. There is a possibility that the drug could significantly help your client, but it is not known if the results, as published in your professional journal, apply to him. The drug is also very expensive. Mr Helm does not know about the new drug. He comes to see you as part of ongoing rehabilitation, and expresses dissatisfaction with the current treatment plan. He wistfully says that he wishes there was something else he could try.

Coordinated care places emphasis on working as a team. In relation to any particular client, the objectives of care, arrived at by the team, are crucial. Discussing what each member of the team is aiming for is important, as is discussed in Chapters 1 and 2 (coordinated care is discussed in Chapter 2).

Libertarian theories, in particular, would allow as much choice as possible to be made by the individual patient. The professional may be obliged to promote such a choice if they adhere to libertarian or other autonomy-based theories. Apart from issues of ability to make treatment and life decisions, apparent in case one, there is an issue of information disclosure here. The professional holds information that may be relevant to the patient's choice. The importance of the patient knowing relevant information before treatment decisions are made is discussed in Chapter 3. Paternalism, which contrasts sharply with libertarianism, may be at work if the practitioner is withholding so much information from the patient that patient choice is effectively nullified.

Deontology would ask whether the possible treatment really is better for this client. Research is essentially a balance of risks and benefits, as discussed in Chapter 9. This is so in drug development and research too as outlined in the section on drugs in Chapter 2. Is a new untried treatment better than the myriad of treatments and side effects currently available to Mr Helm? This value judgement clearly needs to be made with professional clinical expertise and with relevant medical facts available.

In the second case study above, the facts given are scant. If the risks include significant harm, the ethical obligation to care may translate into an obligation to protect rather than chance further injury. The chance of further injury can be hard to predict in situations where complex conditions are treated with multiple powerful drugs. You may like to consider whether you are sufficiently knowledgeable or skilled to deal with that drug, or with the combination of it and other medications that Mr Helm is currently taking (and will, no doubt, continue to take). The limits of skill are a central issue in caring, and this is the subject of a reflective exercise in Chapter 1.

The obligation to provide the best available treatment is double-edged. You may have an idea of what is best, but is it 'available'? Certain utilitarian theories that hold that good should be available to the greatest number give society ethical authority to limit the availability of resources. Under these theories, limiting the access that certain individuals have to certain resources is justifiable if those individuals consume 'too much' of the health care budget.

The next two cases highlight the different approach you can use to begin your analysis, if you make use of the various models of ethics analysis.

Exercise 10.3 Specific requests

CASE THREE

A 15-year-old girl, Karen, who is doing her year 10 exams soon, comes to see a general practitioner. She says she feels tired but can't sleep, and is very worried that she won't do well in her exams. Karen asks for sleeping tablets. She does not want her parents or her normal doctor to know that she is seeking medical treatment.

The most common starting point for ethics analysis is the model suggested by Beauchamp and Childress.[2] You will remember that their principles are beneficence, non-maleficence, autonomy, and justice. When you separate out the issues into these four categories, or try to brainstorm what might be a concern in each of the four, you have made a good start to recognising the complexity of the case. For Karen, autonomy and the decision-making process will loom large. Once you have the issue tagged under autonomy, you can start to identify what is problematic about it. You might look back to the sections on competency and decision making, as in Chapters 3 and 5, or to those of confidentiality in Chapter 4. The purpose of care might be discussed, and you could consider the options that may be open to professionals who see Karen. Just stating the existence of an issue does not solve it. You will need to explore each issue, and discuss if the issues are in conflict: such as if a patient's choice (autonomy) conflicts with the needs and resources available to others (justice).

The ethics theories and frameworks are very helpful in deciding how to resolve conflicts between the shorthand principles.

The Beauchamp and Childress model has appeal partly because of its simplicity, and partly because it can realistically be undertaken by any interested party. Professionals can readily use it. So can patients themselves if they wish, or their family. It is useful for policy makers and administrators too, as it includes big picture issues of resources alongside potential complexities of individual circumstances and situations. It is quite useful in 'macro' community type decisions, as well as 'micro' individual issues.

Two of the other models that have been presented for you are those by Jonsen, Siegler, and Winslade[3], and the rules of thumb by Jennett[4], both included in Chapter 3. These are clinically focused, and seem to be compatible with an analysis undertaken primarily by the clinician.

Exercise 10.4 Care and understanding

CASE FOUR

An 87-year-old man, Mr M, is in a nursing home, in reasonable health for his age apart from forgetfulness of recent events and chronic hip pain. He was admitted after the death of his wife from cancer. The local GP had said Mr M had been about to have hip surgery but postponed it to a few weeks after the funeral. The nursing home is preparing Mr M for the trip to hospital for a hip replacement. Each time the process is explained to him, he forgets by the next day. The operation is booked for one week's time.

What should the nursing home staff do, and why?

If you were to start with Jonsen, Siegler, and Winslade's model, you would first try to understand the 'medical indications', or what the medical situation facing the patient is. Then, you would look for evidence of client preferences, consider quality of life, and finally contextual features like the resources and so on. Notice that you would summarise the issues in a different sequence to that if you were using Beauchamp and Childress's model. Some of the same issues would appear of course. The primary starting point is the health or medical issue to be dealt with, so the process is health carer driven, and seems in that sense to be favouring a carer's view of important features to consider. This is similar to the 'enhanced autonomy' model you read about in relation to decision making (Chapter 3), in which decisions to be made are limited to those judged to be appropriate by the clinician. This seems a sensible emphasis, given that the health professionals are making themselves available to offer benefit to patients.

If you were to apply Jennett's rules of thumb, you are considering whether to apply a specific action or treatment option. So, it is important to identify likely treatment options, and then analyse each one. You would consider whether the proposed treatment is appropriate, or rule it out if it is unnecessary, likely to be unsuccessful, unsafe, unkind, or unwise. Some of these emphasise judgements of care and likely benefit, some emphasise likely harm, and some emphasise issues of resources and justice. So, again, elements that you would discuss if you used Beauchamp and Childress's principles appear in your analysis. Notice again though the emphasis of care issues, and a clinician interpretation of those. There is little explicitly on autonomy built in to this rule of thumb analysis, except that each treatment is an 'option' or choice potentially to be offered to the patient.

As you think about your first reaction to each case, think about the values and concerns that are prominent for you. As you read back over your notes in the book, you should be well on the way to recognising which ethical theories you favour, and to identifying the ethical tools that are useful in your ethical reflection on your health care work. This process of reflection is the start of integrating ethics routinely in your own health care work.

The process of reflection is well suited to groups. If you are working, and have finished your training, you may like to do a few of the exercises with some colleagues in an informal group, or as part of a professional development program. If you are training, you may have a group of colleagues and students around you, in which case you are fortunate enough to have a ready-made group for ethical reflection.

Such groups are usually led by a tutor or lecturer. This book has been written with these teachers of health care ethics in mind. Many of the exercises can be set as individual or group work, and tutorial exercises have been increased in this second edition. It is recommended that teachers work through the book first before they start a teaching program. So many of the issues are interrelated that students may raise concepts that are covered in more detail in later chapters.

A GUIDE TO FURTHER READING

You may like to read further in ethics. Some of the books listed below are geared to particular ethical theories. Most are written for clinical contexts. Some of the books on the list are compilations of the work of different philosophers. A selection of legal references is also included, as ethics and law often work together. All of these references have been referred to in this book.

Annas, G. J., *Judging Medicine*, Humana Press, Clifton, New Jersey, 1988.

Beauchamp, T. L. and Childress, J. F., *Principles of Biomedical Ethics*, 5th edn, Oxford University Press, New York, 2001.

Bennett, B., *Law and Medicine*, Law Book Company Information Services, North Ryde, Sydney, 1997.

Campbell, A., Charlesworth, M., Gillett, G., and Jones, G., *Medical Ethics*, 2nd edn, Oxford University Press, Auckland, 1997.

Charlesworth, M., *Bioethics in a Liberal Society*, Cambridge University Press, Cambridge, 1993.

Collinson, D., *Fifty Major Philosophers: A Reference Guide*, Routledge, London, 1987.

Devereux, J., *Medical Law: Text, Cases and Materials*, Cavendish, Sydney, 1997.

Dix, A., Errington, M., Nicholson, K., and Powe, R., *Law for the Medical Profession in Australia*, 2nd edn, Butterworth Heinemann, Port Melbourne, 1996.

Gillon, R., *Philosophical Medical Ethics*, John Wiley & Sons, Chichester, 1986.

——, (ed.), *Principles of Health Care Ethics*, John Wiley & Sons, Chichester, 1994.

Honderich, T. (ed.), *The Oxford Companion to Philosophy*, Oxford University Press, Oxford, 1995.

Jonas, H., *The Imperative of Responsibility: In Search of an Ethics for the Technological Age*, University of Chicago Press, Chicago, 1984.

Jonsen, A. R., Siegler, M., and Winslade, W. J., *Clinical Ethics: A Practical Approach to Ethical Decisions in Clinical Medicine*, 4th edn, McGraw Hill, New York, 1998.

Mill, J. S., *Three Essays*, Oxford University Press, London, 1975.

Moreno, J. D., *Deciding Together: Bioethics and Moral Consensus*, Oxford University Press, New York, 1995.

Nicholson, R. H., *Medical Research with Children: Ethics, Law, and Practice*, Oxford University Press, Oxford, 1986.

Parker, M. and Dickenson, D., *The Cambridge medical ethics workbook: Case studies, commentaries and activities*, Cambridge University Press, Cambridge, 2001.

Pellegrino, E. D. and Thomasma, D. C., *For the Patient's Good*, Oxford University Press, New York, 1988.

Singer, P., *Practical Ethics*, Cambridge University Press, Cambridge, 1979.

Sullivan, R. J., *Immanuel Kant's Moral Theory*, Cambridge University Press, Cambridge, 1989.

Warnock, M., *Making Babies: Is there a right to have children?*, Oxford University Press, Oxford, 2002.

Summary of key issues

- Theoretical choices and processes of analysis
- Your preferences of tools for your analysis
- Application of analysis to hypothetical cases and real situations

Notes

1 See H. Brody, 'The Four Principles and Narrative Ethics', in R. Gillon (ed.) *Principles of Health Care Ethics*, John Wiley & Sons, Chichester, 1994, p. 211.
2 T. L. Beauchamp and J. F. Childress, *Principles of Biomedical Ethics*, 5th edn, Oxford University Press, New York, 2001.
3 A. R. Jonsen, M. Siegler, and W. J. Winslade, *Clinical Ethics: A Practical Approach to Ethical Decisions in Clinical Medicine*, 4th edn, McGraw Hill, New York, 1998.
4 B. Jennett, 'Quality of care and cost containment in the U.S. and the U.K.', *Theoretical Medicine*, vol. 10, no. 3, 1989, pp. 207–15.

BIBLIOGRAPHY

'Abortion Hero Turns Pro-Life', *Sydney Morning Herald* [reprinted from the *New York Times*], Saturday 12 August 1995, p. 17.

Acute and Co-ordinated Care Branch, Commonwealth Department of Health and Ageing. Primary Care Initiatives: Further Co-ordinated Care Trials. 20 November 2000, at http://www.health.gov.au/hsdd/primcare/acoorcar/abtrials.htm.

Africa News Service, 'Nigerian woman resists deportation', *Africa News Service*, November 21, 2000, p1008325u3785.

Aiken, L. H., Clarke, S. P., Sloane, D. M., Sochalski, J., and Silber, J. H., 'Hospital nurse staffing and patient mortality, nurse burnout, and job dissatisfaction', *Journal of the American Medical Association*, vol. 288, no. 16, 2002, pp. 1987–93.

Alcorn, G., 'Mercy Death World First: Cancer Sufferer First to Die under Northern Territory Euthanasia Law', *Sydney Morning Herald*, Thursday 26 September 1996, p. 1.

Alexandra, A. and Woodruff, A., 'A Code of Ethics for the Nursing Profession', in M. Coady and S. Bloch (eds), *Codes of Ethics and the Professions*, Melbourne University Press, Melbourne, 1996, pp. 226–43.

Andersen, B. and Aranson, E., 'Iceland's database is ethically questionable', *British Medical Journal*, vol. 318, no. 7197, 1999, p. 1565.

Annas, G. J., 'Baby Fae: The "Anything Goes" School of Human Experimentation', *The Hastings Center Report*, vol. 15, no. 1, 1985, pp. 15–16.

——, *Judging Medicine*, Humana Press, Clifton, New Jersey, 1988.

——, 'The Changing Landscape of Human Experimentation: From Nuremberg and Helsinki to AIDS and Cancer', talk given at Grand Rounds, Royal Prince Alfred Hospital, Sydney, Friday 7 August 1992.

Appelbaum, P. S. and Grisso, T., 'Capacities of Hospitalized, Medically Ill Patients to Consent to Treatment', *Psychosomatics*, vol. 38, no. 2, 1997, pp. 119–25.

Asch, D. A. and Ubel, P. A., 'Rationing By Any Other Name', *New England Journal of Medicine*, vol. 336, no. 23, 1997, pp. 1668–71.

Associated Press, AFP, 'Baboon Man out of Hospital', *Weekend Australian*, 6–7 January, 1996, p. 11.

Australian Bureau of Statistics, *Hospitals Australia 1991–92*, Cat. no. 4391.10, Australian Bureau of Statistics, Canberra, 1993.

——, *Private Hospitals 1994–95*, Cat. no. 4390.0, Australian Bureau of Statistics, Canberra, 1996.

Australian Federation of AIDS Organisations (AFAO), Submission to the Baume Review of the Drug Evaluation and Access Process in Australia, May 1991.

Australian Health Ethics Committee and Office of the Federal Privacy Commissioner, Review of guidelines under Section 95 of the Privacy Act 1988, Canberra, April 2003.

Australian Law Reform Commission, 'Background Report No. 22', in Australian Law Reform Commission, *Privacy*, vol. 1, AGPS, Canberra, 1983.

Australian Medical Association (AMA), *AMA Code of Ethics*, AMA, Canberra, 1996

Bacchetti, P. and Moss, A. R., 'Incubation Period of AIDS in San Francisco', *Nature* vol. 338, 1989, pp. 251–3.

Barker, S. F., 'What is a Profession?', *Professional Ethics: A Multidisciplinary Journal* vol. 1, nos. 1&2, 1992, pp. 73–99.

Baume, P., 'Voluntary Euthanasia and Law Reform', *Australian Quarterly*, vol. 68 no. 3, 1996, pp.17–23.

Beauchamp, T. L. and Childress J. F., *Principles of Biomedical Ethics*, 2nd edn, Oxford University Press, New York, 1983.

——, *Principles of Biomedical Ethics*, 3rd edn, Oxford University Press, New York, 1989.

——, *Principles of Biomedical Ethics*, 4th edn, Oxford University Press, New York, 1994.

——, *Principles of Biomedical Ethics*, 5th edn, Oxford University Press, New York, 2001.

Benko, L. B., and Bellandi, D., 'The rough and tumble of it', *Modern Healthcare*, vol. 31, no. 12, 2001, pp. 53–4.

Bennett, B., *Law and Medicine*, Law Book Company Information Services, North Ryde, Sydney, 1997.

Berg, K., 'Ethical Aspects of Early Diagnosis of Genetic Diseases', *World Health*, vol. 5, 1996, pp. 20–1.

Berglund, C. A., 'Australian Standards for Privacy and Confidentiality of Health Records in Research: Implications of the Commonwealth Privacy Act', *Medical Journal of Australia*, vol. 152, 1990, pp. 664–9.

——, 'A Survey of Sydney Adults about the Conduct of Medical Research', *Australian Health Review*, vol. 17, no. 1, 1994, pp. 135–44.

——, 'Children in Medical Research: Australian Ethical Standards', *Child: Care, Health and Development*, vol. 21, no. 2, 1995, pp. 149–59.

——, 'Mandatory HIV Testing of Patients and Professionals: Bringing Ethics into Practice', *Medical Education*, vol. 29, 1995, pp. 360–3.

——, 'Bioethics: A Balancing of Concerns in Context', *Australian Health Review*, vol. 20, no. 1, 1997, pp. 43–52.

——, 'Thoughts Before Whistling', *Australian Health Review*, vol. 20, no. 4, 1997, pp. 5–12.

Berglund, C.A. (ed.), *Health research*, Oxford University Press, Melbourne, 2001.

Berglund, C. and Devereux, J., 'Consent to medical treatment: children making medical decisions for others', *Australian Journal of Forensic Sciences*, vol. 32, 2000, pp. 25–6.

Berglund, C. A. and McNeill, P. M., 'Guidelines for Research Practice in Australia: NHMRC Statement & Professional Codes', *Community Health Studies*, vol. 13, no. 2, 1989, pp. 121–9.

Berglund, C. A., Mitchell, K., and Cox, K., *Exploring Clinical Ethics*, distance module in Masters of Clinical Education course, 2nd edn, University of New South Wales, Sydney, 1993.

Berglund, C. A., O'Brien, E. A., and Magney, A. G., 'Communication and Discussion of Health Research in the Press', platform paper delivered at the Australasian and New Zealand Association for Medical Education Silver Anniversary Conference—Communication: Art and Science; Past and Future; Near and Far, Melbourne, 6–9 July 1997.

Berglund, C. A., Pond, C. D., Harris, M. F., McNeill, P. M., Gietzelt, D., Comino, E., Traynor, V., Meldrum, E., and Boland, C., 'The Formation of Professional and

Consumer Solutions: Ethics in the General Practice Setting', *Health Care Analysis*, vol. 5, no. 2, 1997, pp. 164–7.

Berglund, C. A., Pond, D. C., Traynor, V., Gietzelt, D., McNeill, P. M., Harris, M. F., and Comino, E., 'General Practice and Ethics: Listening and Understanding Concerns Raised by General Practitioners and Consumers', paper presented at the Fifth National Conference of the Australian Bioethics Association, Melbourne, 3–6 April 1997.

Berlant, J. L., *Profession and Monopoly: A Study of Medicine in the United States and Great Britain*, University of California Press, Berkeley, California, 1975.

Berryman, J., 'Discussing the Ethics of Research on Young Children', in J. van Eys (ed.), *Research on Children: Medical Imperatives, Ethical Quandaries, and Legal Constraints*, University Park Press, Baltimore, Maryland, 1978, pp. 85–104.

Blonder, I., 'Blowing the Whistle', in M. Coady and S. Bloch (eds), *Codes of Ethics and the Professions*, Melbourne University Press, Melbourne, 1996, pp. 166–90.

Bolsin, S., 'Professional misconduct: the Bristol case', *Medical Journal of Australia*, vol. 169, 1998, pp. 369–72.

Bossuyt, M. J., *Guide to the 'Travaux Preparatoires' of the International Covenant on Civil and Political Rights*, Martinus Nijhoff Publishers, Dordrecht, 1987.

Brahams, D., 'Right to Know in Japan' [letter], *Lancet*, vol. 2, 1989, p. 173.

Breen, K., Plueckhahn, V., and Cordner, S., 'Medical Registration and Discipline', in *Ethics, Law & Medical Practice*, Allen & Unwin, St Leonards, Sydney, 1997, pp. 77–99.

Brody, H., 'The Four Principles and Narrative Ethics', in R. Gillon (ed.), *Principles of Health Care Ethics*, John Wiley & Sons, Chichester, 1994, pp. 207–15.

Brown, N. 'The "Harm" in Euthanasia', *Australian Quarterly*, vol. 68, no. 3, 1996, pp. 26–35.

Buppert, C., 'Complying with patient privacy requirements', *Nurse Practitioner*, vol. 27, no. 5, 2002, pp. 12–32.

Burnard, P., *Counselling Skills for Health Professionals*, 2nd edn, Chapman & Hall, London, 1994.

Callahan, D., 'Achievable goals', *World Health*, no. 5, 49th year, 1996, pp. 6–8.

Campbell, A., 'Ethics in a bicultural context—a report from New Zealand', *Bioethics*, vol. 9, no. 2, 1995, p. 149–54.

Campbell, A., Charlesworth, M., Gillett, G., and Jones, G., *Medical Ethics*, 2nd edn, Oxford University Press, Auckland, 1997.

Cassarett, D. J., Karlawish, J. H. T., and Moreno, J. D., 'A taxonomy of value in clinical research', *IRB: Ethics & human research*, vol. 24, no. 6, 2002, pp. 1–6.

CCH, 'Death With Dignity', sections 22–268, *Australian Health and Medical Law Reporter*, CCH, Sydney, update regularly.

Centers for Disease Control, 'Revision of the CDC Surveillance Case Definition for Acquired Immunodeficiency Syndrome', *Morbidity and Mortality Weekly Report*, vol. 36, supplement no. 1S, 1987, [inclusive page numbers].

——, 'Public Health Service Statement on Management of Occupational Exposure to Human Immunodeficiency Virus, Including Considerations Regarding Zidovudine Postexposure Use', *Morbidity and Mortality Weekly Report*, vol. 39, no. RR–1, 1990, [inclusive page numbers].

Chalmers, I. and Silverman, W. A., 'Professional and Public Double Standards on Clinical Experimentation', *Controlled Clinical Trials*, vol. 8, no. 4, 1987, pp. 388–91.

Chant, K., Lowe, D., Rubin, G., Manning, W., O'Donoughue, R., Lyle, D., Levy, M., Morey, S., Kaldor, J., Garsia, R., Penny, R., Marriott, D., Cunningham, A., and Tracy, G. D., 'Patient-to-Patient Transmission of HIV in Private Surgical Consulting Rooms' [letter], *Medical Journal of Australia*, vol. 342, 1993, pp. 1548–9.

Charlesworth, M., *Bioethics in a Liberal Society*, Cambridge University Press, Cambridge, 1993.

Cica, N., *The Euthanasia Debate in Australia—Legal and Political Issues*, issues paper no. 2, Australian Institute of Health Law & Ethics, February 1997.

Collins, D. B., 'The Impact of No-Fault Compensation on the Regulation of Medical Practice in New Zealand', *Medicine & Law*, vol. 12, 1993, pp. 61–9.

Collinson, D., *Fifty Major Philosophers: A Reference Guide*, Routledge, London, 1987.

Commission for Health Improvement, *National Patients Survey Programme: 2003 Results*, NHS, London, 2003, at <http://www.chi.nhs.uk/eng/surveys/nps2003>.

Commonwealth Department of Foreign Affairs and Trade, 'Major Step to Protect Rights of Children', *Australian Foreign Affairs and Trade*, vol. 61, no. 12, 1990, p. 893.

Commonwealth Department of Health and Family Services, *Supplement to Medicare Benefits Schedule Book* of 1 November 1996 (effective 1 May 1997), AGPS, 1997.

Commonwealth Department of Human Services and Health, Calls for Expressions of Interest in Conducting Trials in Coordinated Care, Commonwealth Department of Human Services and Health, Canberra, September 1995.

Commonwealth Government of Australia, *National HIV/AIDS Strategy: A Policy Information Paper*, AGPS, Canberra, 1989.

Coney, S., *The Unfortunate Experiment: The Full Story Behind the Inquiry Into Cervical Cancer Treatment*, Penguin, Auckland, 1988.

Connell, J., 'Doctors Seek Powers to Test for HIV', *Sydney Morning Herald*, 5 April 1994, p. 3.

Coombes, R., ''Paternalism' at the root of body parts nightmare', *Nursing Times*, vol. 97, no. 6, pp. 10–11.

Corsino, B. V., 'Bioethics Committees and JCAHO Patients' Rights Standards: A Question of Balance', *The Journal of Clinical Ethics*, vol. 7, no. 2, 1996, pp. 177–81.

Coverdale, J., 'Ethics in Forensic Psychiatry', in W. Brookbanks (ed.), *Psychiatry and the Law: Clinical and Legal Issues*, Brookers, Wellington, 1996, pp. 59–70.

Cox, K., 'Stories as case knowledge: case knowledge as stories', *Medical Education*, vol. 35, 2001, pp. 862–6.

Czecowoski, B. J. A., *Privacy and Confidentiality of Health Care Information*, American Hospital Association, 1984.

Dawson, R. T., 'Drugs in sport—the role of the physician', *Journal of Endocrinology*, vol. 170, no. 1, 2001, pp. 55–61.

Deber, R. B., Kraetschmer, N., and Irvine, J., 'What Role do Patients Wish to Play in Treatment Decision Making?', *Archives of Internal Medicine*, vol. 156, 1996, pp. 1414–20.

De Grazia, D., 'Moving Forward in Bioethical Theory: Theories, Cases, and Specified Principlism', *Journal of Medicine and Philosophy*, vol. 17, 1992, pp. 511–39.

Department of Health and Human Services (DHHS), Guidelines for assessing possible research misconduct in clinical research and clinical trials, DHHS, Rockville, MD, USA, 2001.

de Ridder, D., Depla, M., Severens, P., and Malsch, M., 'Beliefs on Coping with Illness: A Consumer's Perspective', *Social Science & Medicine*, vol. 44, no. 5, 1997, pp. 553–9.

Devereux, J., *Medical Law: Text, Cases and Materials*, Cavendish, Sydney, 1997.

de Vries, B. and Cossart, Y. E., 'Needlestick Injury in Medical Students', *Medical Journal of Australia*, vol. 160, 1994, pp. 398–400.

De Vries, W. C., 'The Physician, the Media, and the "Spectacular" Case', *Journal of the American Medical Association*, vol. 259, no. 6, 1988, pp. 886–90.

Di Angelis, A. J., Born, D. O., and Hill, A. J., 'State Dental Boards and Mandatory HIV Testing', *Northwest Dentistry*, vol. 71, no. 5, 1992, pp. 33–5.

Dickens, B. M., 'Issues in Preparing Ethical Guidelines for Epidemiological Studies', *Law, Medicine & Health Care*, vol. 19, nos. 3–4, 1991, pp. 175–83.

——, 'Legal Approaches to Health Care Ethics and the Four Principles', in R. Gillon (ed.), *Principles of Health Care Ethics*, John Wiley & Sons, Chichester, United Kingdom, 1994, pp. 305–17.

Dickenstein, E., Erlen, J., and Erlen, J. A., 'Ethical Principles Contained in Currently Professed Medical Oaths', *Academic Medicine*, vol. 66, no. 10, 1991, pp. 622–4.

Dickinson, G. M., Morhart, R. E., Klimas, N. G., Bandea, C. I., Laracuente, J. M., and Bisno, A. L., 'Absence of HIV Transmission From an Infected Dentist to His Patients: An Epidemiologic and DNA Sequence Analysis', *JAMA*, vol. 269, no. 14, 1993, pp. 1802–6.

Dix, A., Errington, M., Nicholson, K., and Powe, R., *Law for the Medical Profession in Australia*, 2nd edn, Butterworth Heinemann, Port Melbourne, 1996.

'Doctor Helped Woman Commit Suicide', *Sydney Morning Herald* (reprinted from the *New York Times*), 7 June 1990, p. 12.

'Dolly's Cloners Say No to Families', *Australian*, Friday 27 June 1997, p. 7.

Dorr-Gold, S. and Klipp, G., 'Managed care members talk about trust', *Social Science & Medicine*, vol. 54, no. 6, 2002, pp. 879–88.

Douglas, M., 'Risk Acceptability According to the Social Sciences', *Social Research Perspectives—Occasional Reports on Current Topics*, Russell Sage Foundation, New York, 1985.

Dow, S., 'Trials and Terror: Medical Ethics Under the Microscope', *Sydney Morning Herald*, Saturday 14 June 1997, p. 35.

Doyal, L., 'Clinical ethics committees and the formulation of health care policy', *Journal of Medical Ethics*, vol. 27 Suppl. 1, 2001, pp. 144–9.

Dunne, E., 'Consultation, rapport, and collaboration: essential preliminary stages in research with urban Aboriginal groups', *Australian Journal of Primary Health Interchange*, vol. 6, no. 1, 2000, pp. 6–14.

Dworkin, G., 'Law and Medical Experimentation: Of Embryos, Children and Others with Limited Capacity', *Monash University Law Review*, vol. 13, 1987, pp. 189–206.

Edgar A., 'A Discourse Approach to Quality of Life Measurement', in A. Surbone and M. Zwitter (eds), 'Communication with the Cancer Patient: Information and Truth', *Annals of the New York Academy of Sciences*, vol. 809, 1997, pp. 30–9.

English, V., Roman-Critchley, G., Sheather, J., Sommerville, A., and Dehn, G., 'Would you "blow the whistle"?', *British Medical Journal*, vol. 325, 2002, p. 541.

Faroque, F., 'Impolite Doctors Top List of Complaints', *The Age*, Saturday 7 December 1996, p. A8.

Ferngren, G. B., 'Roman Lay Attitudes Towards Medical Experimentation', *Bulletin of the History of Medicine*, vol. 59, no. 4, Winter, 1985, pp. 495–505.

Finnis, J., 'The Rights and Wrongs of Abortion', in M. Cohen (ed.), *The Rights and Wrongs of Abortion*, Princeton University Press, Princeton, 1974, pp. 85–113.

Finucane, P., Myser, C., and Ticehurst, S., '"Is she fit to sign doctor?"—Practical Ethical Issues in Assessing the Competence of Elderly Patients', *Medical Journal of Australia*, vol. 159, 1993, pp. 400–3.

Flaherty, D. H., *Protecting Privacy in Surveillance Societies*, University of North Carolina Press, Chapel Hill, 1989.

Flew, A., 'The Principle of Euthanasia', in A. B. Downing (ed.), *Euthanasia and the Right to Death*, Nash Publishing, Los Angeles, 1970, pp. 30–48.

Foot, P., 'Killing and Letting Die', in J. L. Garfield and P. Henessey (eds), *Abortion: Moral and Legal Perspectives*, University of Massachusetts Press, Amherst, Massachusetts, 1985, pp. 177–85.

Forrester, K. and Griffiths, D., *Essentials of law for health professionals*, Harcourt, Sydney, 2001.

Foster, P., 'Girl, 15 forced to have new heart', *Sydney Morning Herald*, Saturday 17 July, 1999, p. 19.

Frankel, M. S., 'The Development of Policy Guidelines Governing Human Experimentation in the United States: A Case Study of Public Policy-Making for Science and Technology', *Ethics in Science & Medicine*, vol. 2, 1975, pp. 43–59.

Freckelton, I., 'Enforcement of Ethics', in M. Coady and S. Bloch (eds), *Codes of Ethics and the Professions*, Melbourne University Press, Melbourne, 1996, pp. 130–65.

'Frozen Embryos in Legal Limbo', *Sydney Morning Herald* [reprinted from the *New York Times*], Wednesday 3 June 1992, p. 15.

Fryback, D. G. and Lawrence, W. F., 'Dollars May Not Buy as Many QALYs As We Think: A Problem With Defining Quality-Of-Life Adjustments', *Medical Decision Making*, vol. 17, no. 3, 1997, pp. 277–84.

Gerber, P., 'Has Informed Consent Become a Legal Nightmare?', *Medical Journal of Australia*, vol. 163, 1995, pp. 262–4.

Gert, B., 'Morality, Moral Theory, and Applied and Professional Ethics', *Professional Ethics: A Multidisciplinary Journal*, vol. 1, nos. 1&2, 1992, pp. 5–24.

Gillett, G., 'The New Ethical Committees: Their Nature and Role', *New Zealand Medical Journal*, vol. 102, 1989, pp. 314–15.

Gillon, R., 'Medical Oaths, Declarations, and Codes', *British Medical Journal*, vol. 290, 1985, pp. 1194–5.

——, *Philosophical Medical Ethics*, John Wiley & Sons, Chichester, 1986.

—— (ed.), *Principles of Health Care Ethics*, John Wiley & Sons, Chichester, 1994.

Gilmore, N., 'The Impact of AIDS on Drug Availability and Accessibility', *AIDS*, vol. 5, supplement no. 2, 1992, pp. S253–S262.

Gomez, A. G., Grimm, C. T., Yee, E. F. T., and Skootsky, S. A., 'Preparing residents for managed care practice using an experience-based curriculum', *Academic Medicine*, vol. 72, no. 11, 1997, pp. 959–65.

Grace, D. and Cohen, S., *Business Ethics*, Oxford University Press, Melbourne, 1995.

Grisso, T. and Vierling, L., 'Minors' Consent to Treatment: A Developmental Perspective', *Professional Psychology*, vol. 9, 1978, pp. 412–27.

Hall, M., 'Bush OKs limited stem-cell funding', *USA Today*, Friday 10 August 2001, p. 1.

Hamblin, J., 'Let's Make it Legal: Morality and the Law', paper presented at a meeting on equity and rationing in health, held at the Centre for Values, Ethics and the Law in Medicine, Sydney University, Sydney, 11 November 1996.

Harman, G., 'Moral Relativism Defended', *Philosophical Review*, vol. 84, 1975, pp. 3–22.

Harrison, C. and Laxer, R.M., 'A bioethics program in pediatric rheumatology', *The Journal of Rheumatology*, vol. 27, no. 7, 2000, pp. 1780–2.

Hawkes, N., 'Arthritic Dolly is mutton dressed as lamb', *The Times*, Saturday January 5, 2002, p. 22.

Hawkes, N. and Rhodes, T., 'Human Clones Within Two Years', *Weekend Australian*, 8–9 March 1997, p. 15.

'Health Inequality: The UK's Biggest Issue' [editorial], *Lancet*, vol. 349, 1997, p. 1185.

Heard, S. E., 'Multidisciplinary Response of San Francisco General Hospital to the AIDS Epidemic', *American Journal of Hospital Pharmacy*, vol. 46, 1989, pp. S7–S10.

Henry, D., Keys, C., Balcazar, F., and Jopp, D., 'Attitudes of Community-Living Staff Members Towards Persons with Mental Retardation, Mental Illness, and Dual Diagnosis', *Mental Retardation*, vol. 34, no. 6, 1996, pp. 367–79.

Henry, D. and Lexchin, J., 'The pharmaceutical industry as a medicines provider', *The Lancet*, vol. 360, no. 9345, 2002, pp. 1590–2.

Heussner, R. C. Jr and Salmon, M. E., 'Where Medicine and Media Clash', *Minnesota Medicine*, vol. 72, no. 3, 1989, pp. 141–5.

'HIV Doctor Struck Off', *Daily Telegraph*, Tuesday 26 August 1997, p. 5.

Honderich, T. (ed.), *The Oxford Companion to Philosophy*, Oxford University Press, Oxford, 1995.

Hope, T. and Slowther, A., 'Clinical ethics committee in the UK', *Bulletin of Medical Ethics*, vol. 178, 2002, pp. 13–15.

Horton, R., 'The real lessons from Harold Frederick Shipman', *The Lancet*, vol. 357, 2001, pp. 82–3.

Hoshino, K., 'Information and Self-Determination', *World Health*, vol. 5, 1996, p. 12.

Hubert, E. M., Douglas-Stelle, D., and Bickel, J., 'Context in Medical Education: The Informal Ethics Curriculum', *Medical Education*, vol. 30, 1996, pp. 353–64.

Institute of Medicine (USA), *The AIDS Research Program of the National Institutes of Health*, National Academy Press, Washington DC, 1991.

Jagger, J., Hunt, E. H., Brand-Elnaggar, J., and Pearson, R. D., 'Rates of Needle-Stick Injury Caused by Various Devices in a University Hospital', *New England Journal of Medicine*, vol. 319, no. 5, 1988, pp. 284–8.

James, P. D., *Devices and Desires*, Penguin, London, 1989.

Jennett, B., 'Quality of care and cost containment in the U.S. and the U.K.', *Theoretical Medicine*, vol. 10, no. 3, 1989, pp. 207–15.

Joel, A., 'The Man Who Cares For Kids', *Sydney Morning Herald: Good Weekend*, 4 January 1997, pp. 23–5.

Johnstone, M-J., 'Bioethics and the Wider Community: A Nursing Perspective', *Proceedings of the First Annual Bioethics Association Conference: Bioethics and the Wider Community*, University of Melbourne, 5–7 April 1991, pp. 103–16.

Jonas, H., 'Philosophical Reflections on Experimenting with Human Subjects', *Daedalus*, vol. 98, no. 2, 1969, pp. 219–47.

——, *The Imperative of Responsibility: In Search of an Ethics for the Technological Age*, University of Chicago Press, Chicago, 1984.

Jones, J. H., *Bad Blood: The Tuskegee Syphilis Experiment*, Free Press, New York, 1981.

Jonsen, A. R., Siegler, M., and Winslade, W. J., *Clinical Ethics: A Practical Approach to Ethical Decisions in Clinical Medicine*, 4th edn, McGraw-Hill, New York, 1998.

Kitzhaber, J. and Kemmy, A. M., 'On the Oregon Trail', *British Medical Bulletin*, vol. 51, no. 4, 1995, pp. 808–18.

Kottow, M. H. 'Who is my brother's keeper?', *Journal of Medical Ethics*, vol. 28, 2002, pp. 24–7.

Knultgen, J., *Ethics and Professionalism*, University of Pennsylvania Press, Philadelphia, 1988.

Krugman, S. and Giles, J. P., 'Viral Hepatitis: New Light on Old Disease', *Journal of the American Medical Association*, vol. 212, no. 6, 1970, pp. 1019–29.

Kuhse, H., 'Caution, Not Panic, On Cloning', *Australian*, 12 June 1997, p. 11.

Larriera, A., 'Doctors' HIV: Patients Will Ask', *Sydney Morning Herald*, 3 August 1994, p. 5.

Law Reform Commission of Western Australia, *Medical Treatment For Minors: Discussion Paper*, Law Reform Commission of Western Australia, Perth, 1988.

Lederberg, M. S., 'The Psychological Repercussions of New York State's Do-Not-Resuscitate Law', in A. Surbone and M. Zwitter (eds), *Communication with the Cancer Patient: Information and Truth*, Annals of the New York Academy of Sciences, vol. 809, 1997, pp. 223–36.

Lee, J. W., Director-General Elect, Speech to the Fifty-sixth World Health Assembly, 21 May 2003, Geneva, Switzerland, at http://www.who.int/dg_elect/wha56_jwlspeech/en/print.html.

Leiken, S., 'A Proposal Concerning Decisions to Forgo Life-Sustaining Treatment for Young People', *Journal of Pediatrics*, vol. 115, no. 1, 1989, pp. 17–22.

Le Moncheck, L., 'Philosophy, Gender Politics, and in Vitro Fertilization: A Feminist Ethics of Reproductive Healthcare', *Journal of Clinical Ethics*, vol. 7, no. 2, 1996, pp. 160–81.

Lennane, K. J., 'Whistleblowing: A Health Issue', *British Medical Journal*, vol. 307, 1993, pp. 667–70.

Levine C., Dubler, N. N, and Levine, R. J., 'Building a New Consensus: Ethical Principles and Policies for Clinical Research on HIV/AIDS', *IRB: A Review of Human Subjects Research*, vol. 13, nos 1–2, 1991, pp. 1–17.

Levine, R. J., *Ethics and Regulation of Clinical Research*, Urban & Schwarzenberg, Baltimore and Munich, 1986.

Levitt, M., 'Let the consumer decide? The regulation of commercial genetic testing', *Journal of Medical Ethics*, vol. 27, no. 6, 2001, pp. 398–404.

Liang, B. A., 'The adverse event of unaddressed medical error: identifying and filling the holes in the health-care and legal systems', *Journal of Law, Medicine & Ethics*, vol. 29, 2001, pp. 346–68.

Lo, B., 'Clinical Ethics and HIV Illnesses', *Medical Care Review*, vol. 47, no. 1, 1990, pp. 15–32.

Lockwood, M., 'When Does a Life Begin', in M. Lockwood (ed.), *Moral Dilemmas in Modern Medicine*, Oxford University Press, London, 1985, pp. 9–31.

Lovell, R., 'Ethics At the Growing Edge of Medicine: The Regulatory Side of Medical Research', *Australian Health Review*, vol. 9, no. 3, 1986, pp. 234–50.

Lustig, B. A., 'The Method of "Principlism": A Critique of the Critique', *Journal of Medicine and Philosophy*, vol. 17, 1992, pp. 487–510.

Lyall, K., '30-baht health care a fatal prescription', *The Australian*, Wednesday April 24, 2002, p. 8.

McBride, G., 'Living Liver Donor', *British Medical Journal*, vol. 299, 1989, pp. 1417–18.

McCombs, J. S. [letter], *New England Journal of Medicine*, vol. 335, no. 19, 1996, p. 1465.

McDowell, B., 'The Excuses that Make Professional Ethics Irrelevant', *Professional Ethics: A Multidisciplinary Journal*, vol. 3, nos 3&4, 1994, pp. 157–70.

MacLeod, P. and Clarke, F. F., 'Forget cloning and pay attention to China', *Canadian Medical Association Journal*, vol. 159, no. 2, 1998, pp. 153–5.

McNeill, P. M., 'The Implications for Australia of the New Zealand Report of the Cervical Cancer Inquiry: No Cause for Complacency', *Medical Journal of Australia*, vol. 150, 1989, pp. 264–96.

McNeill, P. M., Walters, J. D., and Webster, I. W., 'Ethical Issues in Australian Hospitals', *Medical Journal of Australia*, vol. 160, 1994, pp. 63–5.

Magney, A. G. and Berglund, C. A., 'Co-ordinated care: ethics debate as part of the trial process', *Evaluation*, vol. 6, no. 4, 2000, pp. 455–69.

Malley, B., 'Professionalism and Professional Ethics', in D. E. Edgar (ed.), *Social Change in Australia*, Cheshire, Melbourne, 1974, pp. 391–408.

Mallon, D. F. J., Shearwood, W., Malla, S. A., French, M. A. H., and Dawkins, R. L., 'Exposure to Blood Borne Infections in Health Care Workers', *Medical Journal of Australia*, vol. 157, 1992, pp. 592–5.

Marcus, R., 'Surveillance of Health Care Workers Exposed to Blood From Patients Infected With Human Immunodeficiency Virus', *New England Journal of Medicine*, vol. 319, 1988, pp. 1118–23.

Marino, K., *Resumes for the Health Care Professional*, John Wiley & Sons, New York, 1993.

Marquet, R. L., Bartelds, A., Visser, G. L., Spreeuwenberg, P., and Peters, L., 'Twenty five years of requests for euthanasia and physician assisted suicide in Dutch general practice: trend analysis', *British Medical Journal*, vol. 327, no. 7408, 2003, p. 201–2.

Medical Council of Canada, 'CLEO: Objectives of the Considerations of the Legal, Ethical and Organizational Aspects of the Practice of Medicine', Medical Council of Canada, Ottawa, Ontario, 1999.

Medical Records Association of Australia, *Code of Ethics*, Medical Records Association, Canberra, undated.

Medical Research Council, 'The Ethical Conduct of Research on Children', *Bulletin of Medical Ethics*, vol. 96, 1992, pp. 8–9.

Milio, N., 'The Press and Policy-Making: Clues for Creating a Health-Promoting Climate', *International Quarterly of Community Health Education*, vol. 10, no. 4, 1989–90, pp. 329–45.

Mill, J. S., 'On Liberty', in J. S. Mill, *Three Essays*, Oxford University Press, London, 1975, pp. 92–114.

Mitchell, K. R. and Lovat, T. J., *Bioethics for Medical and Health Professionals*, Social Sciences Press, Wentworth Falls, New South Wales, 1991.

Momber, J. M. and Rueda, R. M., 'Bioethics and Medical Practice', *World Health*, 49th year, 1996, no. 5, pp. 29–31.

Moodie, A-M., 'A Code of Ethics Doesn't Ensure Business Ethics', *Australian Financial Review*, Friday 18 July 1997, p. 61, quoted in S. Cohen and D. Grace, *Business Ethics*, Oxford University Press, Melbourne, 1995.

Mooney, G. H., Russell, E. M, and Weir, R. D, *Choices for Health Care: A Practical Introduction to the Economics of Health Provision*, 2nd edn, Macmillan, London, 1986.

Moreno, J. D., *Deciding Together: Bioethics and Moral Consensus*, Oxford University Press, New York, 1995.

Morris, P., 'County dental care is in crisis', *Gloucestershire Echo*, Friday July 18, 2003, pp. 1–2; P. Morris, 'Queueing for NHS dentists—is it Prestbury next?', *Gloucestershire Echo*, Wednesday July 30, 2003, p. 3.

Morrow, L., 'When One Body Can Save Another', *Time*, 17 June 1991, pp. 46–50.

Motor Accidents Authority, *NSW Health Bulk Billing Handbook*, State Health Publications No. (FB) 960105, Motor Accidents Authority, Sydney, May 1996.

Mulhall A., 'Anthropology, Nursing and Midwifery: A Natural Alliance?', *International Journal of Nursing Studies*, vol. 33, no. 6, 1996, pp. 629–37.

Murphy, T. F., 'Physician-Assisted Suicide and the Slippery Slope', *Department of Medical Education Bulletin*, vol. 3, no. 2, 1996, p. 1.

Nakajima, H., 'Health, Ethics and Human Rights', *World Health*, no. 5, September–October, 49th Year, 1996, p. 3.

National Commission for the Protection of Subjects of Biomedical and Behavioral Research, *Report and Recommendations: Institutional Review Boards*, Department of Health, Education and Welfare publication no. (OS) 78-0008, United States Government Printer, 1978.

National Health and Medical Research Council, *The Media and Public Health: A Discussion of the Role of the Media in Promoting the Health of the Public*, (Standing Subcommittee on Health Promotion and Education, and Subcommittee on the Media and Health Promotion), NHMRC, Canberra, August 1984.

——, 'The National Health and Medical Research Council and Ethical Regulation: A Short History', *Australian Health Review*, vol. 9, no. 3, 1986, pp. 234–8.

——, Communicating with patients: advice for medical practitioners. Draft document, as at 2003.

——, *National Statement on Ethical Conduct in Research Involving Humans*, Canberra, AGPS, 1999.

——, *Human Research Ethics Handbook: Commentary on the National Statement on Ethical Conduct in Research Involving Humans*, endorsed 25 October 2001, Canberra, AGPS, 2002.

New South Wales Department of Health (Audit Branch), 'Hospital Booking List Clinical Priority Classification System (93/57)', in *Patient Matters: Manual for Area Health Services and Public Hospitals*, New South Wales Department of Health, Sydney, June 1989 (updated regularly), section 12.11.

——, 'Health Records and Information: Policies 81/218', in *Patient Matters: Manual for Area Health Services and Public Hospitals*, Sydney, June 1989, section 9.

New South Wales Medical Board, *2002 Annual Report*, Gladesville, 2002.

Newton, J. S., Ard, W. R., Horner, R. H., and Toews, J. D., 'Focusing on Values and Lifestyle Outcomes in an Effort to Improve the Quality of Residential Services in Oregon', *Mental Retardation*, vol. 34, no. 1, 1996, pp. 1–12.

New Zealand Medical Association Newsletter, no. 108, 1994, p. 3.

Nicholson, R. H., *Medical Research with Children: Ethics, Law, and Practice*, Oxford University Press, Oxford, 1986.

——, 'Bioethics Attacked in Germany' (editorial review), *Bulletin of Medical Ethics*, vol. 61, 1990, pp. 19–23.

Noonan, J. T., 'An Almost Absolute Value in History', in J. Feinberg (ed.), *The Problem of Abortion*, Wadsworth, Belmont, California, 1973, pp. 10–17.

O'Brien, E., 'Making a note and handover', Chapter 10 pp. 113–34, in C. Berglund and D. Saltman, *Communication for health care*, Oxford University Press, Melbourne, 2002.

Oliver, J. and Webb, D. J., 'Sildenafil for "blue babies". Such unlicensed drug use might be justified as last resort', *British Medical Journal*, vol. 325, no. 7373, 2002, p. 1174.

Olsen, D. P., 'Populations Vulnerable to the Ethics of Caring', *Journal of Advanced Nursing*, vol. 18, 1993, pp. 1696–700.

Oosterhof, J. E. J., Scholten-Linde, J. L. J., Houtepen, R., and Berglund, C. A., 'The Interpretation of Morality: Cross-Purposes in the Australian Euthanasia Debate', unpublished paper.

Otlowski, M., *Implications of genetic testing for Australian Insurance Law and Practice*, Occasional Paper No. 1, Centre for Law and Genetics, University of Tasmania Law School, University of Melbourne Faculty of Law, Hobart and Parkville, 2001.

Parker, M. and Dickenson, D., *The Cambridge medical ethics workbook: case studies, commentaries and activities*, Cambridge University Press, Cambridge, 2001.

Parliament of New South Wales, 'Budget Paper No. 3 Vol. 2', Budget Estimates 2002–03, Parliamentary Paper No. 97b of 2002, ordered to be printed 4 June 2002.

Patterson, Senator the Hon. Kay, Minister for Health and Ageing. Media Release. *A fairer Medicare—better access, more affordable.* April 28, 2003.

Peabody, J. W., Bickel, S. R., and Lawson, J. S., 'The Australian Health Care System: Are the Incentives Down Under or Right Side Up?', *JAMA*, vol. 276, no. 24, 1996, pp. 1944–50.

Pearson, S. D., Sabin, J. E., and Hyams, T., 'Caring for patients within a budget: physicians' tales from the front lines of managed care', *Journal of Clinical Ethics*, vol. 13, no. 2, 2002, pp. 115–23.

Peel, P., 'Community participation in decision-making and service delivery', *Canberra Bulletin of Public Administration*, vol. 94, 1999, pp. 34–51.

Pellegrino, E., 'The metamorphosis of medical ethics: A 30 year retrospective', *Journal of the American Medical Association*, vol. 269, no. 9, 1993, pp. 1158–62.

Pellegrino, E. D., 'Character, Virtue and Self-Interest in the Ethics of the Professions', *Journal of Contemporary Health Law and Policy*, vol. 5, 1989, pp. 53–73.

Pellegrino, E. D., and Thomasma, D. C., *For the Patient's Good: The Restoration of Beneficence in Health Care*, Oxford University Press, New York, 1988.

Pennisi, E. and Williams, N., 'Will Dolly Send in the Clones?', *Science*, vol. 275, 1997, pp. 1415–16.

Pincus, R. C., 'Has Informed Consent Finally Arrived in Australia?', *Medical Journal of Australia*, vol. 159, 1993, pp. 25–7.

Plomer, A., 'Beyond the HFE Act 1990: The regulation of stem cell research in the UK', *Medical Law Review*, vol. 10, 2002, pp. 132–64, at p. 133.

Pratt, J., 'Redefining the Core Values and Role of General Practice in the UK', *Education for Health*, vol. 10, no. 1, 1997, pp. 35–45.

Price, V. and Roberts, D. F., 'Public Opinion Processes', in C. R. Berger and S. H. Chaffee (eds), *Handbook of Communication Science*, Sage, Newbury Park, California, 1987, pp. 781–816.

Qiu, R-Z., 'Bioethics in an Asian Context', *World Health*, vol. 5, 1996, pp. 13–15.

Queensland Law Reform Commission, *Assisted and Substituted Decisions: Decision-Making By and for People with a Decision-Making Disability*, report no. 49, vol. 1, Queensland Law Reform Commission, Brisbane, June 1996.

Quill, T. E., and Brody, H., 'Physician Recommendations and Patient Autonomy: Finding a Balance Between Physician Power and Patient Choice', *Annals of Internal Medicine*, vol. 125, no. 9, 1996, pp. 763–9.

Rachels, J. A., 'Active and Passive Euthanasia', *New England Journal of Medicine*, vol. 5, 1975, pp. 39–45.

Ramsay, S., 'Audit further exposes UK's worst serial killer', [news] *The Lancet*, vol. 357, 2001, pp. 123–5.

Ramsey, P., 'The Enforcement of Morals: Non-Therapeutic Research on Children', *Hastings Center Report*, vol. 6, no. 4, 1976, pp. 21–30.

Rawls, J., *A Theory of Justice*, Belknap Press, Harvard, 1971.

Redfern, M., Keeling, J. W., and Powell, E., *The Royal Liverpool Children's Inquiry, Summary & Recommendations*, The Stationery Office, London, 30 January 2001.

Reuter, 'Hospital Faker Ends in Doc', reprinted in *Sydney Morning Herald*, Saturday 30 December 1995, p. 10.

Richardson, J., 'The Importance of Perspective in the Measurement of Quality-Adjusted Life Years', *Medical Decision Making*, vol. 17, no. 1, 1997, pp. 33–41.

Robotham, J., 'Thigh gives heart a leg-up and offers alternative to stem cells', *Sydney Morning Herald*, Thursday 9 May 2002, p. 3.

Rocker, G. M., Cook, D. J., Martin D. K., and Singer, P. A., 'Seasonal bed closures in an intensive care unit: a qualitative study', *Journal of Critical Care*, vol. 18, no. 1, 2003, pp. 25–30.

St Vincent's *Bioethics Newsletter*, vol. 1, no. 3, 1983, p. 12.

Schlink, L., 'Dolly dies of lung disease', *Sunday Telegraph*, 16 February 2003, p. 40.

——, 'New baby from dead husband', *Sunday Telegraph*, 10 February 2002, p. 46.

Schneider, G. W. and Snell, L., 'C.A.R.E.: an approach for teaching ethics in medicine', *Social Science & Medicine*, vol. 51, no. 10, 2000, pp. 1563–7.

Scott, J., 'Syringe May Have Held Virus: QC', *The Australian*, 30 August 1994, p. 3.

Shooner, C., 'The Ethics of Learning From Patients', *Canadian Medical Association Journal*, vol. 156, no. 4, 1997, pp. 535–8.

Singer, P., *Practical Ethics*, Cambridge University Press, Cambridge, 1979.

Singh, K. and Gan, G. L., 'An Asian Perspective on Euthanasia', *Australian Quarterly*, vol. 68, no. 3, 1996, pp. 36–45.

Skene, L., 'What Should Doctors Tell Patients?', *Medical Journal of Australia*, vol. 159, 1993, pp. 367–8.

Slaytor, E. and Lesjak, M., 'Euthanasia Seminar', *In the News* (Newsletter of the New South Wales Branch of the Public Health Association), vol. 11, no. 2, 1997, p. 7.

Smith & Nephew Surgical, *Hospital and Health Services Year Book 1995/96*, 20th edn, Peter Isaacson Publications Pty Ltd, Prahran, Victoria, 1996.

Smith, D., 'Human genome project', *Sydney Morning Herald*, 27 February 2003, pp. 23–4.

——, 'Cloning study points to early end for Dolly', *Sydney Morning Herald*, Monday 11 February, 2002, p. 6.

Smith, J., 'The Shipman Inquiry. Third Report: Death Certification and Investigation of Deaths by Coroners.' Presented to Parliament by the Secretary of State for the Home Department and the Secretary of State for Health by Command of Her Majesty July 2003. Cm5854. Whitehall, London, July 2003.

Smith, L. F. P. and Morrissy, J. R., 'Ethical Dilemmas for General Practitioners Under the UK New Contract', *Journal of Medical Ethics*, vol. 20, 1994, pp. 175–80.

Solomon, W. D., 'Rules and Principles', in W. T. Reich (ed.), *Encyclopedia of Bioethics*, vol. 1, The Free Press, New York, 1978, pp. 407–13.

Sorlier, V., Forde, R., Lindseth, A., and Norberg, A., 'Male physicians' narratives about being in ethically difficult care situations in paediatrics', *Social Science & Medicine*, vol. 53, no. 5, 2001, pp. 657–67.

Spark, M., *Memento Mori*, Penguin, Middlesex, 1959.

Spencer, S., 'AIDS: Some Civil Liberty Implications', in P. Byrne, *Ethics and Law in Health Care and Research*, John Wiley & Sons, Chichester, 1990.

Spicker, S. F., Alon, I., de Vries, A., and Engelhardt, H. T. Jr, *The Use of Human Beings in Research*, Philosophy and Medicine 28, Kluwer Academic Publishers, Dordrecht, 1988.

Staff reporters, 'Troubled transplant man throws in bad hand', *The Australian*, Monday February 5, 2001, p. 5.

Sullivan, R. J., *Immanuel Kant's Moral Theory*, Cambridge University Press, Cambridge, 1989.

Surbone, A., 'Truth-Telling, Risk, and Hope', in A. Surbone and M. Zwitter, *Communication with the Cancer Patient: Information & Truth*, Annals of the New York Academy of Sciences, vol. 809, New York Academy of Sciences, New York, 1997, pp. 72–9.

Suzuki, D. and Knudtson, P., *Genethics: The Ethics of Engineering Life*, Allen & Unwin, Sydney, 1989, pp. 345–6.

Taerk, G., Gallop, R. M., Lancee, W. J., Coates, R. A., and Fanning, M., 'Recurrent Themes of Concern in Groups for Health Care Professionals', *AIDS Care*, vol. 5, no. 2, 1993, pp. 215–22.

Taylor, H. A. and Kass, N. E., 'Attending to local justice: lessons from pediatric HIV', *IRB: Ethics & human research*, vol. 24, no. 6, 2002, pp. 9–17.

Tegtmeier, J. W., 'Ethics and AIDS: A Summary of the Law and Critical Analysis of the Individual Physician's Ethical Duty to Treat', *American Journal of Law & Medicine*, vol. 16, nos 1–2, 1990, pp. 249–65.

Thomson, C., 'Personnel', in *CCH Australian Health & Medical Law Reporter*, (looseleaf service), updated regularly, pp. 6–400.

Thomson, J. J., 'A Defense of Abortion', *Philosophy and Public Affairs*, vol. 1, no. 1, 1971, pp. 47–66.

Todd, A. M., Lacey, E. A., and McNeill, F., "I'm still waiting...': barriers to accessing cardiac rehabilitation services', *Journal of Advanced Nursing*, vol. 40, no. 4, 2002, pp. 413–20.

Tomaszewski, T., 'Ethical Issues From an International Perspective', *International Journal of Psychology*, vol. 124, 1979, pp. 131–5.

Tooley, M., 'Abortion and Infanticide', in J. Feinberg (ed.), *The Problem of Abortion*, Wadsworth, Belmont, California, 1973, pp. 51–91.

Ubel, P. A., DeKay, M. L., Baron, J., and Asch, D. A., 'Cost-Effectiveness Analysis in a Setting of Budget Constraints', *New England Journal of Medicine*, vol. 334, no. 18, 1996, pp. 1174–7.

United Nations, 'International Covenant on Civil and Political Rights', in M. J. Bossuyt, *Guide to the 'Travaux Preparatoires' of the International Covenant on Civil and Political Rights*, Martinus Nijhoff Publishers, Dordrecht, 1987.

United States Department of Health, Education, and Welfare, *Ethical Principles and Guidelines for the Protection of Human Subjects of Research* [The Belmont Report], United States Department of Health, Education, and Welfare, Washington DC, 1978, (Department of Health, Education, and Welfare publication no. OS 78–0012).

——, *Federal Register*, vol. 43, no. 9, Friday 13 January 1978, pp. 4110–18.

——, Privacy Rule, Federal Regulations, vol. 67, no. 157, 14 August 2002, pp. 53181–273.

Urbina, C., Kaufman, A., and Derksen, D., 'The Managed Health Care Scenario: Challenges to Future Medical Training', *Education for Health*, vol. 10, no. 1, 1997, pp. 25–33.

Veatch, R. M., *Cross Cultural Perspectives in Medical Ethics*, Jones and Bartlett Publishers, Boston, 1989.

——, 'Justice in Health Care: The Contribution of Pellegrino', *Journal of Medicine and Philosophy*, vol. 15, 1990, pp. 269–87.

Vinten, G., 'Whistle While You Work in the Health Related Professions?', *Journal of the Royal Society of Health*, vol. 114, no. 5, 1994, pp. 256–62.

Walker, J., Lyall, K., and Hawes, R., 'Wooldridge Backs Inquiry on Guinea-Pig Babies', *The Australian*, Wednesday 11 June 1997, pp. 1, 2.

Wall, S. D., Olcott, E. W., and Gerberding, J. L., 'AIDS Risk and Risk Reduction in the Radiology Department', *American Journal of Roentology*, vol. 157, no. 5, 1991, pp. 911–17.

Walsh, M., *The National Childhood Immunisation Campaign—Ethical Issues: Topics for Attention*, Issues Paper No. 3 (Autumn 1997), The Australian Institute of Health Law & Ethics, 1997.

Warnock, M., 'Do Human Cells Have Rights?', *Bioethics*, vol. 1, no. 1, 1987, pp. 1–14.

Warnock, M., *Making babies: is there a right to have children?*, Oxford University Press, Oxford, 2002.

Weeramantry, C. G. and Giantomasso, D. F., *Consent to the Medical Treatment of Minors and Intellectually Handicapped Persons*, Faculty of Law, Monash University, Melbourne, 1983.

Westin, A. F., *Privacy and Freedom*, Atheneum, New York, 1970.

Williams, M. V., Parker, R. M., Baker, D. W., Parik, N. S., Pitkin, K., Coates, W. C., and Nurss, J. R., 'Inadequate Functional Literacy Among Patients at Two Public Hospitals', *JAMA*, vol. 274, no. 21, 1995, pp. 1677–82.

World Health Organization, *Basic Documents*, 26th edn, World Health Organization, Geneva, 1976.

——, 'Documentation Requirements for Approval: Safety', *WHO Drug Information*, vol. 10, no. 4, 1996, pp. 180–1.

——, 'Drug Safety Monitoring Centres', *WHO Drug Information*, vol. 10, no. 4, 1996, p. 181.

——, Alert, verification and public health management of SARS in the post-outbreak period, 14 August 2003. At <http://www.who.int/csr/sars>.

World Medical Association, Declaration of Helsinki 1964 (as revised at the 35th World Medical Assembly, Venice 1983), World Medical Association, 1983.

——, 'WMA to continue discussion on Declaration of Helsinki', Press release, 14 September 2003, at <http://www.wma.net>.

Yarborough, M., Jones, T., Cyr, T. A., Phillips S., and Stelzner, D., 'Interprofessional education in ethics at an academic health sciences center', *Academic Medicine*, vol. 75, no. 8, 2000, pp. 793–800, at p. 794.

Young, T., 'Teaching Medical Students to Lie', *Canadian Medical Association Journal*, vol. 156, no. 2, 1997, pp. 219–22.

Zeleznik, D., Habjanic, A., and Micetic Turk, D. M., 'Teaching ethics to students in the University College of Nursing Studies in Maribor', *Medicine and Law*, vol. 19, no. 3, 2000, pp. 433–9.

Zwart, H., 'Rationing in the Netherlands: the Liberal and Communitarian Perspective', *Health Care Analysis*, vol. 1, no.1, 1993, pp. 53–6.

INDEX